how happy is your Health?

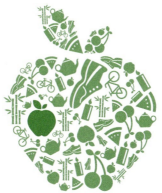

50 Great Tips to Help You Live a Long, Happy and Healthy Life

Sophie Keller

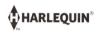

How Happy Is Your Health?
ISBN-13: 978-0-373-89247-1

© 2011 by Sophie Keller

All rights reserved. The reproduction, transmission or utilization of this work in whole or in part in any form by any electronic, mechanical or other means, now known or hereafter invented, including xerography, photocopying and recording, or in any information storage or retrieval system, is forbidden without the written permission of the publisher. For permission please contact Harlequin Enterprises Limited, 225 Duncan Mill Road, Don Mills, Ontario, Canada, M3B 3K9.

Author photograph by Sarah Corwin Photography
Illustrations by Serena Zanello

The health advice presented in this book is intended only as an informative resource guide to help you make informed decisions; it is not meant to replace the advice of a physician or to serve as a guide to self-treatment. Always seek competent medical help for any health condition or if there is any question about the appropriateness of a procedure or health recommendation.

A full list of references used in writing this book can be found at www.HowHappyIs.com

Library of Congress Cataloging-in-Publication Data
Keller, Sophie.
  How happy is your health? : 50 great tips to help you live a long, happy and healthy life / Sophie Keller.
       p. cm.
Includes bibliographical references.
ISBN 978-0-373-89247-1 (hardback)
1. Health. 2. Well-being. 3. Happiness. I. Title.
RA776.K2817 2011
613—dc22
                              2011010357

How Happy Is is a trademark of Sophie Keller.

® and TM are trademarks owned and used by the trademark owner and/or its licensee. Trademarks indicated with ® are registered in the United States Patent and Trademark Office, the Canadian Trade Marks Office and/or other countries.

www.Harlequin.com

Printed in U.S.A.

To my dear friend and healer
Dr. William Hitt (1932-2010) who made
a difference to so many people's lives,
including my own.

CONTENTS

Introduction — ix
Quiz: How Happy Is Your Health? — 1

1 Take Charge of Your Own Health — 9

PART I: HEALTHY EATING — 11

2 Drink Enough Water for *Your* Body — 12
3 Buy Organic—and Know the "Dirty Dozen" — 14
4 Eat These Top 10 Vegetables — 16
5 Eat These Top 10 Fruits — 19
6 Buy the Healthiest Kind of Chicken and Eggs — 22
7 Eat Grass-Fed Beef — 24
8 Avoid Soy for These 4 Reasons — 26
9 Eat Sustainable, Safe Fish — 27
10 Achieve Your Ideal Weight with These Easy and Unusual Tricks — 29
11 Get Rid of Cravings — 31
12 Eat More Raw Food — 33
13 Alkalinize Your Body to Prevent Disease — 35
14 Take Digestive Enzymes — 37
15 Avoid These Food Additives — 38

16	Keep Your Colon Happy	40
17	Choose Sweeteners That Are Good for You	42
18	Take D₃ Supplements	44
19	Take the Right Kind of Supplements	46
20	Get These Essential Vitamins and Minerals	48

PART II: HEALTHY SELF — 53

21	Look Younger from the Inside Out	54
22	Stop These 3 Energy-Draining Habits	56
23	Express Your Feelings for Good Health	58
24	Listen to Calm Music and Sounds to Alleviate Stress	60
25	Embrace Your Age	61
26	Listen to Your Body	63
27	Use Your Language to Help You Lose Weight	65
28	Stay Calm and Stress Free with These Easy Solutions	67

PART III: HEALTHY BODY — 69

29	Combat the Winter Blues with These Simple Tips	70
30	Exercise for Innumerable Benefits	73
31	Practice Pilates for a Lean, Strong and Flexible Body	75
32	Practice Yoga for Excellent Health	77

33	Be Smart about Antibiotics	79
34	Practice Reflexology on Yourself	80
35	Get a Regular, Inexpensive Massage	83
36	Meditate	85
37	Do Acupuncture	88
38	Use Acupressure for Common Ailments	90
39	See a Chiropractor for Back Pain	93
40	Do the Alexander Technique	95
41	Stock Your Homeopathic Medicine Cabinet	97
42	Do Traditional Chinese Medicine	99
43	Use Fluoride-Free Toothpaste and Mouthwash	101
44	Buy Toxin-Free Cosmetics	103
45	Get Beautiful, Natural Nails	105

PART IV: HEALTHY EARTH — 107

46	Avoid BPAs	108
47	Know Which Plastics Are Safe to Use	110
48	Use Your Cell Phone Safely	113
49	Clean Your Home Naturally—and Healthily	116
50	Improve Your Indoor Air Quality	118

Quiz Answers: So, How Happy *Is* Your Health? — 121

Acknowledgments — 129

INTRODUCTION

Your health is number one. That's it. End of story! You can have a great marriage, a great career and a great family but taking care of your health has to come before everything else.

When it comes to your health, you need to think long-term. The question you need to ask yourself is, "how will the way I treat my body now affect it five years, ten years and forty years from now?" If how you are taking care of your body now will support your long-term vitality and help slow down your aging, then go for it, otherwise you need to change some habits before it's too late.

This book provides fifty unusual and original health tips that are easy to implement and have the capacity to make a big impact on the quality of your life. If you follow them, I promise you they will help prevent disease and assist you to live to a ripe old age! My goal is to give you knowledge so that you can make your own informed choices and decide what is best for you.

There are four sections in the book. In the Healthy Eating section you will learn about your food. You will discover which specific fruits and vegetables are important to eat organic, what terms like "free-range" really mean on your egg cartons and easy and unusual ways to achieve your ideal weight.

In the Healthy Self section you will learn about the powerful mind-body connection: how to release anger and express your feelings to make you look younger, how your language can help you lose weight and which three energy-draining habits you will want to do away with.

In the Healthy Body section you will discover alternative healing practices and new ways to exercise, including easy ways to combat the winter blues, which pressure point you can use to help cure a hangover and how changing your posture can change your life.

In the Healthy Earth section you will learn easy ways to avoid common toxins. You will gain an understanding of which specific plastics are safe to use and which are not, why fluoride-free toothpaste is better for you and reasons why you might want to improve the water quality in your home.

My personal health journey began at a very young age. When I was fourteen, I hurt my back and shoulder while playing competitive tennis. I was in excruciating pain and had problems sitting and standing. I went to a host of medical doctors, who said they couldn't help me and insisted I would never be better. As a result, I took my healing into my own hands and explored holistic and drug-free therapies. I did Pilates to strengthen the muscles in my back, started meditating to release stress and clear my mind and went to therapy to understand why my back, "my support system," had given up on me. After seeing the incredible results I could get naturally, I began a lifelong journey to discover more about optimum health and how to achieve it.

Over the years, I realized, among other things, that it is probably better to eat fruits and vegetables that have not been sprayed with poison, that the mind and body are completely intertwined—when one is suffering, the other often follows suit—and that it is a good idea to treat my body as if it is my best friend, since we'll be spending a lifetime together.

I studied under many different doctors at the forefront of complementary medicines and trained in numerous different bodyworks, mind therapies and spiritual practices to heal myself and to gain insight in the field of personal development and happiness. I became a life coach, master practitioner and trainer in neuro-linguistic programming (NLP) and hypnosis, as well as a qualified yoga teacher. Bringing together the knowledge that I gained over the years, I eventually became an expert in the field of happiness.

I've taken many things that I've learned about health and distilled them into these simple and easy to follow tips. I promise that if you follow them it will make a big difference in how you look and feel.

I wish you a long, healthy and happy life.

Love, Sophie

QUIZ: HOW HAPPY IS YOUR HEALTH?

Read each question and circle the answer that best applies to you and your health. If there are steps you can take to improve your health based on your answers, turn to the relevant tips in the book and start creating a happier, healthier and longer life, one tip at a time!

Circle the answer that sounds most accurate, then turn to page 121 for your results.

1. **If you are near a landline and someone calls you on your cell phone, do you:**
   A. Talk on your cell phone without worrying about the time spent on it?
   B. Ask if you can call him or her back from the landline?
   C. Talk on your cell phone but minimize the amount of time you stay on your cell?

2. **Are you aware of the quality of the water that you drink?**
   A. Not at all, and I'm not particularly concerned about it.
   B. I do my best to know about the quality of the water that I drink.

C. I sometimes think about it, but it doesn't influence my choices too much.

3. **When you buy cleaning products for your home, do you:**
    A. Buy the cheapest products you can find?
    B. Think about what would be good for your health and the environment?
    C. Go for whatever catches your eye first?

4. **When it comes to body care and beauty products, do you:**
    A. Look for the most natural and organic brand?
    B. Look for a brand you recognize?
    C. Look for the cheapest brand you can find?

5. **When you use plastic products, are you careful to limit your exposure to potential toxins?**
    A. No, I am not aware of toxins in plastic and don't really think about them.
    B. Yes, I am aware of toxins and try to lessen the amount of plastic products I use and choose them carefully.
    C. I think about this sometimes, but I don't let it influence my choices too much.

6. **When you have an injury or common illness, how do you go about healing it?**
   A. I go straight to my medical doctor and ask for the quickest solution, whether it's a pain pill, antibiotic or some other therapy.
   B. I make lifestyle changes to try to holistically treat the ailment before going to see alternative health practitioners and medical doctors.
   C. I ignore the injury or cold and hope it will go away on its own.

7. **How is your posture?**
   A. Excellent. I'm very careful about my posture and always sit or stand up straight.
   B. I never really think about my posture and have no idea.
   C. Sometimes I think that I could sit or stand straighter.

8. **Are your moods affected by the seasons?**
   A. No, I am not very moody, and I maintain the same general mood all year round.
   B. I tend to get more depressed and moody in the winter.
   C. I can get moody, but it doesn't correlate to any time of the year.

9. How often do you exercise?

   A. I am too busy and rarely have time to exercise, but I try to fit a workout in when I can.

   B. I like to commit to working out at least three times a week.

   C. I don't enjoy exercise and wouldn't be caught dead in a gym!

10. When it comes to diets, are you:

   A. On them intermittently with little long-term success?

   B. Never on a diet as you are happy with your weight?

   C. Always on one diet or another, and often experimenting with new fad diets?

11. Do you treat your body as:

   A. Your best friend?

   B. A separate object, to be used and abused?

   C. A fair-weather friend? You love it when it's in great condition and dislike it when it's not in top form.

12. How do you handle stress?

   A. I find that even the little things stress me out and it's very difficult for me to unwind.

B. I don't easily get stressed about anything.

C. Sometimes I stress and sometimes I don't, but it really depends on the issue.

13. How often do you feel happy?

A. I feel happy no matter what, whether I have or haven't achieved my goals.

B. I feel happy temporarily when I reach a new goal or milestone.

C. I never feel happy—no matter what I accomplish or do.

14. How easily do you express your anger?

A. I find it really easy to express my anger.

B. I tend to hold my feelings in, without expressing them.

C. Sometimes I can express my anger and sometimes I bottle it all in.

15. Do you make food choices based on:

A. How the food will taste the second it is in your mouth, no matter how good or bad it is for you?

B. How the food will feel in your stomach and body in the hours after you have eaten?

C. How the food will fuel your body, but often give in to cravings for sweet and salty foods?

16. When it comes to choosing vitamin and mineral supplements, do you:

A. Tend to buy the cheapest ones on the shelf?

B. Select brand names that you recognize?

C. Choose those that are closest to the food source?

17. How often do you buy organic fruits and vegetables?

A. I go out of my way to buy organic as much as I can, particularly for certain foods.

B. I don't buy organic. It's way too expensive.

C. I sometimes buy organic if it's available, but I don't worry too much about it.

18. When you reach for a snack, do you select:

A. A healthy snack, such as fruits or vegetables or nuts, that will fill you up and give you energy?

B. A treat that satisfies your cravings for sweet, salty or fattening foods?

C. Whatever you're in the mood for at the time, whether it's healthy or not?

19. Are you aware of the quality of animal products that you buy?

A. Yes, I am careful to buy high-quality animal products from humane and healthy sources.

B. I try to buy quality animal products, but I get confused about what all the labels mean.

C. No, I don't want to spend extra for "high-quality" animal products—after all, meat is meat.

20. Which most accurately reflects your regular diet:

A. I'm a meat-and-potatoes kind of person. You'll rarely see a vegetable on my plate!

B. I eat a variety of raw fruits and vegetables, with limited amounts of high-quality animal products, like fish, chicken and beef.

C. I tend to eat whatever is quick and easy, whether it's deli fare, takeout or frozen dinners.

1 Take Charge of Your Own Health

Even though we now have access to advanced Western medicine and have so many amazing choices when it comes to health care, good health does not start with your doctor. It starts with you!

Your body is completely different from anyone else's, and if you listen to it, you will know it better than any doctor ever could. Not understanding how your body works is like not opening your mail for fear of what you might find. With the same verve with which you study your favorite hobby, you need to understand how your mind and body work separately and synergistically.

You and your body are together for a lifetime, and if you look after it, it will look after you. Take good care of your body—eat right, stay active and limit your levels of stress. If your body is trying to tell you something through pain or illness, do not ignore it or get frustrated that it is "letting you down."

We all have health conditions or issues due to our genetics and lifestyle. Perhaps you are prone to stomach upset, have a low thyroid, are susceptible to anemia, have high blood pressure or intermittently suffer from a back problem. The important thing is to know your body and what your issues tend to be.

Once you pinpoint your health conditions, you can do your own research, weigh all your treatment options and choose which approach or combination of approaches works best for you. It makes sense to start with the most holistic and natural therapies and go from there. And don't think you need to wait until you're in a crisis to take care of yourself. It is better to see a professional at the first sign of back pain than to wait until your back is thrown out to get help! Whenever possible, catching warning signs early on is the way to go and will make your recovery that much easier.

Always remember that your health is in your hands. You control how you take care of your body every day. And when you get sick, you decide how you want to go about healing yourself. This book is full of ideas to get you started. Love your body, look after it, nurture it with the love and care you had or would have liked to have had as a child and you'll find that, over time, it will return the favor and treat you really well, too.

PART I

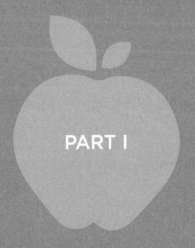

HEALTHY EATING

2 Drink Enough Water for *Your* Body

Your body is up to 70 percent water. Every system in your body depends on water. Water flushes toxins out of the organs, carries nutrients to the cells and provides a moist environment for ear, nose and throat tissues. When you don't drink enough water to carry out those functions, dehydration occurs, which can drain your energy and, in the long term, prevent your body from functioning properly.

So how much water should you really drink? That depends on the climate in which you live, your body weight and how active you are. If you live in a hot climate, exercise vigorously on a regular basis or are suffering from an illness, then you need to drink more water. A common rule of thumb is to drink eight eight-ounce glasses of water a day. Or you can drink as many ounces of water as half your weight. Caffeine and alcohol do not count toward your daily intake as they are dehydrating. Neither do sports or soft drinks that contain sugar. The true litmus test is your urine: if it is clear, then you know that you are drinking enough!

Here are some other points to keep in mind when it comes to drinking water:

1. Drinking water from a plastic water bottle is not good for you because many plastics release toxins. (See tips #46 and #47 for more information.)
2. Get your water supply tested at home to make sure you aren't ingesting chemicals or impurities from your water supply or because of the poor worn away pipes. Look at the clarity of your water, the smell of it and the taste. If it looks cloudy or has an off taste, you want to have it tested. Or you can simply put a filter on your tap or use another common filtration system. Make sure that you filter your tap water before you drink it or cook with it.
3. Learn to love the taste of water. If you want to flavor it, then add a few slices of cucumber, lemon, lime or orange.
4. Make sure that you always have water wherever you go.
5. Make sure that your diet is composed mainly of vegetables and fruits, which are filled with water.

3 Buy Organic—and Know the "Dirty Dozen"

The closer you get to eating food in its natural, raw organic state—whether it's fruits and vegetables or dairy products—the more nutrients you will ingest and the healthier you will be.

Organic Farming

The word *organic* refers to the way farmers grow and process vegetables and fruits and raise animals for human consumption. Organic farmers don't use chemicals or conventional methods to fertilize crops, control weeds or prevent plant disease and instead apply natural fertilizers, such as manure or compost. Nonorganic pesticides are not allowed to be used, including insecticides, fungicides and herbicides, and only certain organic pesticides are allowed. In contrast, conventional farming methods include the use of chemical herbicides to manage weeds, insecticides to reduce pests and disease and chemical fertilizers to promote plant growth. Conventionally raised farm animals are given antibiotics, growth hormones and medications to make them grow quicker and to prevent disease.

Organic farming tends to promote healthy soil and water conservation and reduces pollution. Crop rotation is often practiced to keep essential nutrients in the soil. Instead of being cooped up in small spaces and raised with unnatural feed, drugs and hormones, in organic farming the animals in most cases graze healthfully in pastures.

So buy organic when you can. One of the best places to get fruits, vegetables and many dairy products is at your local farmers' market.

Here is a list of the top twelve fruits and vegetables containing the most pesticides when conventionally grown, according to the Environmental Working Group, a nonprofit research group based in Washington, D.C. You can lower your pesticide consumption quite dramatically by avoiding these contaminated fruits and vegetables and buying their organic counterparts instead.

Organic Fruits and Vegetables to Buy

Apples	Grapes (imported)	Peaches
Bell Peppers	Lettuce	Potatoes
Blueberries	Kale/Collard Greens	Spinach
Celery	Nectarines (imported)	Strawberries

4 Eat These Top 10 Vegetables

If you want to keep your health in tip-top condition, eat vegetables as they are packed with nutrients that your body needs to live a long and healthy life.

Here is a list of the top ten vegetables that I consider essential to maintaining good health. If you eat these ten on a regular basis, you'll be getting a fantastic variety of essential nutrients. These vegetables are best for you when eaten organic and raw. And don't shy away from the variety of colors here. The more colorful your plate looks with natural ingredients, the more likely you are to get a wide range of nutrients.

1. **Spinach:** This is one of the most nutrient-packed foods and is loaded with vitamins and minerals, including iron, vitamin C, beta-carotene, calcium and vitamin K, which is vital for the absorption of calcium.

2. **Broccoli:** This is an incredible super food with cancer-fighting power. Packed full of nutrients, broccoli is very high in calcium, vitamin C and folic acid and can help prevent heart disease.

3. **Sweet Potatoes:** Even though they are called "potatoes," sweet potatoes are not actually related to the potato at all. The antioxidant properties of sweet potatoes can help rid the body of free radicals, which are linked to many chronic illnesses. They also have anti-inflammatory properties. Sweet potatoes are really high in fiber, beta-carotene, vitamin A, potassium, iron and calcium. One study showed that eating sweet potatoes can lower LDL cholesterol by as much as 29 percent. And eating two servings a week can potentially cut your risk of suffering a heart attack by as much as 86 percent.

4. **Onions:** Onions have antiviral, anti-inflammatory and antibiotic properties. They contain powerful antioxidants, promote stomach health and are great for building strong bones.

5. **Kale:** Kale has more nutrient value per calorie than most vegetables. It is packed full of vitamins and minerals, like calcium, iron and vitamins A, C and K.

6. **Collard Greens:** One cup of collard greens provides the same amount of calcium as a glass of milk! They have a huge amount of phytochemicals, which are known to fight cancer, and are packed with fiber, potassium, vitamins A, C, E and K, beta-carotene, magnesium and phosphorous.

7. **Carrots:** Carrots are really high in carotenoids, an antioxidant that has been associated with a lower incidence of

many different types of cancers. Carrots are also known to help strengthen your vision and are also essential for a healthy colon.

8. **Asparagus:** Asparagus contains a huge amount of fiber and vitamin B_6. It also has high levels of folate and potassium.

9. **Garlic:** Garlic is one of the oldest medicinal vegetables. It can reduce plaque and lower cholesterol and is known to decrease the risk of stomach and colon cancer. It also has antiviral, antiparasitic, antibacterial and blood-thinning properties.

10. **Sea Vegetables:** There are a number of different sea vegetables, including arame, nori, wakame, kombu, hijiki and kelp. They are packed full of minerals, vitamins and amino acids and are known to be particularly high in iodine, calcium and iron. Sea vegetables are known to detoxify the body and they have anticancer properties.

5. Eat These Top 10 Fruits

There are many benefits to eating fruit. Aside from being packed with vitamins and minerals, many fruits act as a natural laxative and can regulate digestion. The phytonutrients in fruit (which impart colors to it) are powerful antioxidants. Antioxidants have antiaging properties and can help prevent cancer. These ten fruits have a huge range of vitamins and nutrients, and you would do well to include them in your diet as much as you can. Fruit is generally high in sugar, so be mindful of that if you have to watch your blood sugar levels.

1. **Apples:** Apples are great snack food and are low in calories. You will want to eat them with their skin on as almost half of the vitamin C content is just under the skin. Apples are great for preventing cholesterol buildup, arteriosclerosis and heart disease. They are also a great source of insoluble fiber.

2. **Coconuts:** Coconuts are one of the most beneficial foods you can eat. They help with metabolism and digestion. Coconuts contain fatty acids called medium-chain triglycerides (MCT), which are very easy to metabolize and are used mostly for

energy rather than stored as fat. They also have antiviral and antibacterial properties.

3. **Avocados:** Avocados are great if you want to lower your cholesterol and protect your prostate. The monounsaturated fat in avocados reduces the risk of cancer and diabetes. They are packed full of antioxidants and also are a great source of fiber and potassium. Avocados contain high levels of folate, vitamin A, beta-carotene and other carotenoids.

4. **Blueberries:** Blueberries are the most nutrition-packed berries. They have an abundance of antioxidants. They possess anti-inflammatory properties and help with vitamin absorption. Blueberries are also very rich in vitamins, minerals and fiber.

5. **Bananas:** Studies have shown that the potassium in bananas can boost your learning capabilities. They can prevent elevated blood pressure and the high fiber in bananas helps forestall cardiovascular disease. Bananas are loaded with vitamin B_6 and vitamin C, are rich in fiber and contain amino acids.

6. **Cherries:** Cherries are loaded with powerful anti-inflammatory, antiaging and anticancer compounds. They contain significant amounts of melatonin, a hormone produced in the pineal gland that is known to slow the aging process. Cherries are loaded with vitamins, antioxidants and fiber.

7. **Kiwis:** Kiwis are rich in antioxidants and phytonutrients. They are the most nutrient dense of all the fruits and are exceptionally high in vitamin C. Kiwis are one of the top low-sodium, high-potassium foods. In many studies, kiwis have been shown to prevent cellular damage and even repair damage already done. They are also exceptional as a blood thinner.

8. **Papayas:** Papayas are excellent for digestive health and are often used in digestive enzyme supplements. They contain fiber and folate, which help prevent colon cancer, as well as other diseases.

9. **Grapes:** The skin of grapes contain resveratrol, which researchers think is one of the best potential antiaging substances around. Resveratrol is also known to reduce the risk of cancer and cardiovascular disease and to act as a powerful antioxidant. Grapes are really high in vitamins and minerals.

10. **Cantaloupe:** Over 90 percent of cantaloupe is water, and it is very low in calories, making it a great snack. It is high in vitamin C and vitamin A. Cantaloupe is also known to boost immunity, fight infections, reduce blood pressure and cut cancer risks.

6 Buy the Healthiest Kind of Chicken and Eggs

Eggs are loaded with vitamins and are one of the highest sources of protein, containing all nine essential amino acids. However, it can be really difficult to decipher which eggs are best to buy. Here's a rundown of some common egg labels and what they mean. (This list of labels can also be applied to buying chicken.)

Here are my most recommended to my least recommended eggs:

Pastured: The hens are raised in their natural habitat, in pastures, with access to the sun, grass and bugs and their naturally omnivorous diet may be supplemented with organic grains and other nonchemical feed.

Vegetarian: The hens are fed a vegetarian diet.

Organic: This means that the laying hens are fed organic feed that must not contain chemicals.

Free-Range: In theory, free-range hens have access to an outdoor space, but some egg producers apply the term too loosely, using it if the chickens have access to a *door* to an outdoor area, regardless of how small the area actually is.

Cage Free: The hens are allowed to move around inside the barn and are not housed in cages. However, they are still in a very confined space.

Conventional: The hens have less than half a square foot each, not even enough room to spread their wings.

The labels "Farm Fresh" and "All Natural" mean nothing. The terms are unregulated.

If you want to buy quality eggs, your first stop is pastured eggs as the chickens are raised in their natural environment and, as a result, all the nutrients they enjoy enrich their eggs and, in turn, you.

As I mentioned, these labels can apply to chicken as well. Chicken is a really good source of protein, and it contains many essential vitamins and minerals. But because of the stressful and cruel treatment of conventionally raised chickens and the fact that they are loaded with toxins, antibiotics, steroids, pesticides and growth hormones used in factory farming, I recommend that you avoid eating conventionally grown chicken. Instead, purchase pastured organic chicken, if you can find it.

7. Eat Grass-Fed Beef

When you eat animal products, it's very important to know where they come from and how the animal was fed and treated. It's disturbing to hear that the animal was abused or fed an unnatural diet, and it's important to realize that these conditions can affect the quality of the meat. Most of the meat in supermarkets comes from factory-farmed animals: the animals are fed an unnatural diet, are given antibiotics, are abused and mistreated and are under constant duress. These unhealthy conditions make for unhealthy meat. In stark contrast, grass-fed beef is much better for you.

Here are five other reasons why you need to eat grass-fed meat:

1. The cows are fed grass, which is their natural food, rather than genetically modified grain and soy, which are fed to cows in factory farms. Grass-fed meat is not the same as organic meat. The "organic" label just means that the cows were fed organic grain rather than grass.

2. Farmers who raise grass-fed cows avoid using chemicals, hormones and anything else that makes the cows grow quickly. The animals are raised in healthier, less stressful conditions so they do not need antibiotics. If you eat conventional meat, you ingest all the chemicals, hormones and antibiotics that the factory-farmed cows were given.

3. Grass-fed meat has much less fat, less cholesterol and fewer calories than its factory-farmed, grain-fed counterparts. It is also packed full of nutrients: it has more omega-3 fatty acids, which prevent heart disease, as well as more vitamins A, C and E, and a higher level of CLA (conjugated linoleic acid), which reduces fat accumulation in the body and is known to have cancer-fighting properties.

4. Grass-fed cattle ranchers focus on keeping the grass and land healthy. They know that if the quality of the grass is excellent, the animals eating it will be as well.

5. Grass-fed cows are in their natural habitat and thus generate much less environmental pollution. Factory farms produce a huge amount of waste and this waste frequently ends up in rivers and streams, and ultimately in the water supply.

8 Avoid Soy for These 4 Reasons

Soy protein products come in many different shapes and textures and are falsely marketed to us as health food. But soy products are not actually healthy. Here are four reasons why:

1. Soy contains plant estrogens called phytoestrogens that disrupt hormone function and have been shown to potentially increase the risk of breast cancer.

2. Soy suppresses your thyroid and is known as a goitrogen, a substance that prevents your thyroid from getting the necessary amount of iodine.

3. Soy contains enzyme inhibitors called phytates, which block mineral absorption in the digestive tract.

4. Soy is rich in trypsin inhibitors, which interfere with protein digestion and can cause many digestive problems.

If you do eat soy, make sure you eat small amounts of it and only fermented forms, such as miso, tempeh and soy sauce, as fermentation makes the nutrients in soy more soluble.

9 Eat Sustainable, Safe Fish

Fish is a very important part of a healthy diet and is the best source of omega-3s, as well as containing other essential nutrients. However, overfishing has become the biggest threat to marine wildlife and many fish species are critically endangered. Each one of us can directly discourage overfishing by buying fish that are in abundance and sustainable. You also want to avoid eating fish with high levels of contaminants, especially mercury. Mercury has been found to affect brain development and the nervous system.

Here is a guide from the Natural Resources Defense Council (NRDC):

Eat

- Arctic Char
- Atlantic Mackerel
- Barramundi
- Herring
- Jellyfish
- Mullet
- Mussels
- Oysters
- Pacific Halibut
- Pollock
- Rainbow Trout
- Sablefish
- Sardines
- Squid

Eat Occasionally

This seafood is okay to eat occasionally depending on where it is caught and whether it is farmed or not.

Abalone *(farmed only)*

Anchovy *(avoid North Atlantic and Mediterranean)*

Catfish *(avoid farmed in Asia)*

Clams *(farmed only; avoid canned, Arctic and Atlantic Surf)*

Cod *(Pacific only)*

Crab *(avoid Russian)*

Haddock *(avoid trawled)*

Lobster *(Atlantic only)*

Mahi Mahi *(troll or hook-and-line only)*

Marlin *(avoid Atlantic)*

Octopus *(avoid imported)*

Rockfish

Salmon *(wild Alaskan only)*

Scallops *(U.S. farmed only, avoid Atlantic Giant)*

Shrimp *(avoid foreign farmed, trawled and tiger)*

Snapper *(hook-and-line caught Yellowtail only)*

Striped Bass *(wild Atlantic only)*

Swordfish *(beware of mercury)*

Tilapia *(domestic only)*

Avoid

Atlantic Cod

Atlantic Halibut

Atlantic Sole

Chilean Sea Bass

Dogfish

Grouper

Monkfish

Orange Roughy

Shark

Skate

Tilefish

Tuna *(including Toro)*

10 Achieve Your Ideal Weight with These Easy and Unusual Tricks

It doesn't have to be difficult or complicated to achieve your optimum size. Here are three uncommon pieces of advice to help make it easy.

1. **Put a mirror on your fridge.** This will help you to catch a glimpse of yourself each time you open it and make you aware of how many times you do so unconsciously, as a habit, when you're not even hungry. The mirror makes you do a double take and gives you a second's gap between the cause (stress, boredom) and the response (mindlessly opening the fridge to comfort eat), to help you make a new, healthier decision.

2. **Think before you eat.** Before you put food in your mouth, take a moment to do this exercise: imagine how the meal or snack will feel in your body for the next few hours as it digests. For example, if you have something healthy, like vegetables and lean protein or complex carbs, very likely you will feel energetic for hours and you will feel full until your next meal or healthy snack. However, if you load yourself up

with empty calories like chips, cookies or lots of bread, you will tend to feel heavy and tired for hours after—and you will probably feel hungry again before too long. Remember that food is fuel. You are eating to live, not living to eat. This means becoming conscious of how your body feels in the long term, rather than focusing on things that provide short-lived instant gratification, such as junk food.

3. **Phase out unhealthy foods.** Rather than trying to give up your favorite foods cold turkey, phase them out gradually. Start by writing a list of all the junk food that you eat. Let's say, for example, that your vices are chocolate, chips, French fries, bread and ice cream. Eliminate one vice from your diet at a time, taking at least two weeks to break the habit. For example, if you start with chocolate, find a healthy substitute for it like fresh fruit. After two weeks of sticking to it, you'll find that the cravings will disappear and then, and only then, do you move on to eliminate your next vice. In this way, you are gradually changing your lifestyle and building healthy new habits without feeling deprived. The key is to be patient and consistent, and before you know it the pounds will be dropping off.

11 Get Rid of Cravings

Cravings can be the worst health saboteurs. Most of us crave unhealthy foods, like sweet or salty snacks, which can undo all our efforts to eat well and stay on track. The good news is that it is possible to beat cravings. Here's how.

The key is to find out what your trigger foods are. We all have these foods—the snack that, once you start eating, almost makes you unconscious, since you can't stop until you discover that it's too late and you have eaten the whole chocolate cake, box of cookies or bag of chips. Pinpoint your trigger foods and avoid them as much as possible.

Here are four ways to deal with cravings:

1. Keep the unhealthy food that you crave out of the house so that it is less accessible. Replace the unhealthy food with a similar, but healthier option for when cravings strike. Interestingly, sugar cravings will often subside when you consume protein. If you really crave something sweet, then make sure that you have fruit in the house, and eat fruit the next time a craving strikes.

2. If you're milling around the house or kitchen, craving a food that you know you really shouldn't eat, change your physiology. Go for a walk, even if it's just around the block, or go and work out. The change in physiology can alter your mood and cut cravings.

3. If you are looking for comfort food because you are feeling low or upset, find another way to handle your emotions. Speak to your partner, a friend or a family member. This will help you get the feelings off your chest, and the conversation and human connection will boost your mood much better than chocolate cake ever could.

4. Try sucking on a strong mint, as mint often takes away the desire for food.

12 Eat More Raw Food

The raw food diet is based on eating whole, unprocessed, uncooked foods that are preferably organic. It has been shown to have innumerable health benefits.

Our bodies are made up of over a thousand different types of enzymes and each does a specific job. Without enzymes we cannot breathe, see, move or digest our food. Enzymes keep us alive: they are components of every cell and are found in every tissue of every organ in our body. Enzymes are produced by our bodies, but raw food is also full of natural enzymes that can help support digestion. Since enzymes are very sensitive to heat, most of them are destroyed by cooking, making raw fruits and vegetables much more nutritious and easier to digest than cooked ones. For food to be considered raw, it should not be heated over 116 degrees F.

Here are seven more reasons why you might want to eat a mainly raw food diet:

1. Raw foods encourage weight loss.
2. Raw foods can heal many diseases.

3. The digestive enzymes in raw foods aid digestion.
4. Bacteria and other microorganisms in raw food affect the immune system and digestion by populating the digestive tract with beneficial gut flora.
5. Raw foods have a higher nutrient value than cooked food.
6. Raw foods are high in antioxidants and can slow aging.
7. Raw foods prevent harmful toxins from building up in the body—toxins that cause chronic disease and other problems.

A completely raw food diet is not for everyone. It is generally considered inappropriate for children and pregnant and nursing women, and is also not recommended for those with anemia or those at risk of osteoporosis. If you go on a raw food diet, you need to make sure that you get sufficient calcium, iron, B_{12} and protein.

Even if you don't adopt an entirely raw food diet, you can still reap the benefits by eating more raw foods, like raw fruits, vegetables and nuts, and by avoiding processed foods. Try it out and see how your body feels!

13 Alkalinize Your Body to Prevent Disease

You might remember the concept of acid and alkaline substances from your school science classes. The pH scale ranges from 1 to 14, with 7.0 being neutral, anything from 7.1 to 14 being alkaline and anything from 6.9 to 0 being acidic. Our blood pH level is naturally slightly alkaline, in the range of 7.35 to 7.45.

The different foods you eat can create more alkalinity or acidity in the body. Alternative health practitioners believe that eating a more alkaline diet positively influences the pH of the body and prevents disease and the effects of aging. A diet high in acid-producing foods puts a huge amount of pressure on the body, as it will naturally try to maintain the correct pH of the blood at all costs. The extra effort that the body has to put in can deplete it of alkaline minerals, such as sodium, potassium, magnesium and calcium, making you prone to disease. If you want to determine your pH level, buy some pH strips at a pharmacy and test your saliva or urine.

The acidity and alkalinity levels of a food are based on how that food is assimilated after digestion. For instance, you would think that lemons would be acidic, but actually they are alkaline forming once they are digested in the body.

Alkaline-forming foods include most fruits, green vegetables, peas, beans, lentils, spices, herbs and seasonings, and seeds and nuts. Acidic foods include meat, fish, poultry, eggs, grains, legumes, sugars, coffee, tea, alcohol and processed food (along with emotional stress, toxic overload and too little exercise).

In order to stay healthy and keep disease at bay, it is important to consume a large amount of alkaline-forming foods, like fresh fruits and vegetables, in order to balance the intake of protein and other acidic foods.

An alkaline diet of fruits, vegetables, whole grains, beans, other legumes and healthy oils, such as olive oil and flaxseed oil, allows the body to maintain a slightly alkaline pH, work efficiently and stay healthy. The goal is to eat at least 60 percent alkaline foods and 40 percent, at the most, acidic foods. If you are ill in any way, shift your diet to one that is 80 percent alkaline and 20 percent acid to help you heal.

14 Take Digestive Enzymes

Not only does the kind of food that you eat have an influence in keeping your weight stable, but so does your ability to properly digest your food. Digestive enzymes that are created in the mouth, the stomach and the small intestine break down the food nutrients into simpler forms so that the body can use the food for energy, instead of storing it as fat. The younger you are and the healthier you are, the more enzymes you will have, so the goal is to keep as many enzymes as you can, for as long as you can, by eating as healthily as you can. Raw food contains its own enzymes that aid in digestion (see tip #12); however, as soon as you cook food it kills off enzymes and is harder to digest. That is why it is often a good idea to take a digestive enzyme supplement when you are eating a more complex cooked meal with many different food groups, as the additional supplement will take the pressure off your own enzymes and help you digest. In addition, protein and carbs require different enzymes so you might want to try eating them in separate meals. This will also help with stabilizing your weight.

15 Avoid These Food Additives

Food additives have been used for centuries to preserve flavor and to enhance the taste and appearance of food. However, additives do not add any nutritional value to food and many are very unhealthy. Here are just a few common additives to avoid:

1. **Monosodium Glutamate (MSG/E621):** MSG is used as a flavor enhancer. Adverse affects include depression, headaches, fatigue and weight gain, as it disengages the function in your brain that registers when you're satiated. MSG is found in processed foods like frozen dinners, lunch meats, cookies, chips and so on.

2. **Aspartame (E951):** This artificial sweetener is sold under such brand names as Nutrasweet and Equal. It is found in many foods that are labeled "diet" or "sugar free." Aspartame is believed to be a neurotoxin and carcinogen and is known to create a wide variety of ailments, including dizziness, headaches and mental confusion.

3. **High-Fructose Corn Syrup:** This is a highly refined artificial sweetener that is found in processed foods, bread, candy,

soda and many other products. It is the number one source of calories in the United States. In addition to causing weight gain if eaten in excess, high-fructose corn syrup increases cholesterol levels and the risk of diabetes.

4. **Common Food Dyes:** Avoid food with artificial colors, like tartrazine (E102) and sunset yellow (E110), which can be found in American cheese, candy, sodas and sports drinks. Thought to contribute to behavioral problems in children and to a lower IQ, red dye #3 (E124) was banned in 1990 from use in foods and cosmetics, but it is still on the market until supplies run out. It is found in maraschino cherries, candy, baked goods and ice cream.

5. **Sodium Nitrate/Sodium Nitrite (E250):** Sodium nitrate is a preservative that is added to processed meats. The chemical enhances the color of meat and helps it look fresh longer. The USDA tried to ban it in the late 1970s but was overridden by the meat industry, which protested that it had no alternative for preserving packaged meat products.

6. **Sulfur Dioxide (E220):** This is a preservative used in vitamins, minerals, enzymes and fatty acids. The FDA has prohibited its use on raw fruits and vegetables. Adverse reactions to sulfur dioxide include bronchial problems and hypotension (low blood pressure), and it is not recommended for children.

16 Keep Your Colon Happy

Your colon is an important part of your digestive tract. Its main function is to help absorb water and minerals and to help clear waste from your body. It also contains bacteria that aid digestion and promote vital nutrients to maintain a healthy pH balance and prevent an increase in harmful bacteria. In order to keep your body as healthy and youthful as possible, it's important to keep your colon in good working order! Here are five very simple ways you can do so:

1. Start the day with a glass of warm water or some herbal tea to flush out your system, followed by breakfast to wake up your system.

2. Many people have allergies to common foods like dairy, wheat and eggs without even knowing it. Determine which foods cause you indigestion, gas or diarrhea. All you have to do is practice trial and error. For instance, if you fear you have allergies to wheat, eat some wheat bread or pasta and notice if you have an adverse reaction. If you find that you are irritated by these common foods, avoid them or minimize

your consumption and, as an added bonus, you will probably lose a few pounds as well!

3. Eat more grains, cereals, legumes, nuts, seeds, fruits and vegetables, and avoid processed food and refined sugars, or anything that is unnatural or man-made. The planet supplies everything you need to stay healthy and to give you energy. "Fake" foods don't give you energy; they take energy away and are very difficult to digest.

4. Do your best to avoid eating protein (such as fish, meat, eggs) and carbohydrates (such as bread, potatoes, pasta) in the same meals. Your stomach uses different digestive enzymes to break down carbs than it does for protein, and eating fewer food groups at a time helps digestion and gives you more energy.

5. Take digestive enzyme supplements if you know you are going to eat a rich meal or one that mixes protein and carbohydrates to help you digest better.

17 Choose Sweeteners That Are Good For You

You would be surprised at the amount of hidden sugar that you eat every day. This is because sugar is not just found in candy, but also in microwavable foods, condiments and most packaged foods. As a result, most of us are unconsciously addicted to sugar. This is a problem as not only does sugar store as fat, it also suppresses the immune system—a good reason to stay off sugar if you are ill and want to recover quickly!

If you have no intention of giving up your sweet tooth, then instead of substituting with artificial sweeteners that are packed full of toxic chemicals, choose from some of these healthier options and remember to consume any type of sugar in moderation:

Stevia: This is a calorie-free, natural alternative sweetener and a great substitute for sugar in your tea and coffee.

Raw Honey: Raw honey contains lots of antioxidants, can beautify the skin and is good for digestion. It is high on the glycemic index so it is not so great if you are diabetic or are trying to lose weight.

Agave Syrup: This extract has a similar consistency to honey and tastes sweeter than sugar. It has many health benefits, including boosting the immune system and helping your body absorb many nutrients.

Date Sugar: This extract made from dehydrated dates contains many beneficial minerals. Date sugar is a great natural substitute for sugar in recipes, but it is not ideal for diabetics.

Xylitol: This is a naturally occurring sugar alcohol found in many fruits and vegetables. It can usually replace sugar cup for cup. Xylitol is low on the glycemic index.

Evaporated Cane Juice: Evaporated cane juice is derived from sugar cane, but since only water is removed from the process of refining, it retains all its vitamins and minerals. It is very good for healthy baking!

Fruit Spreads: These concentrated fruit juice syrups are a perfect alternative to jams and other preserves. Fruit spreads contain natural and unrefined fructose. Double check the label to make sure that the spread is not sweetened with sugar.

18 Take D_3 Supplements

Determining the vitamins and minerals that you need to take all depends on your diet and your own particular deficiencies. However, regardless of your diet there is one vitamin that is essential for anyone who does not live in a climate that has sun year-round or who works indoors most of the time: vitamin D_3.

Despite the name, vitamin D_3 is actually not a vitamin; it is a hormone. Research into vitamin D_3 tells us that it is much more essential to our health than we ever realized.

Studies have shown that people who are more likely to get depressed have lower levels of vitamin D_3 and also that a lack of vitamin D_3 can increase the chances of getting a more serious illness, including cancer. Unfortunately, most people are deficient in this essential hormone.

Here are three ways that you can get natural (not synthetic) D_3:

1. **Make sure you have sufficient exposure to the sun.** The optimum is to get fifteen to twenty minutes a day on 40 percent of your body, with no sunscreen! This may not be possible

year-round depending on where you live. And, of course you need to be careful about skin cancer, but if you avoid the sun altogether, you can't benefit from a vital source of nutrition in the sun's rays. You don't want to overexpose yourself to the sun, but you do need it, so find a balance.

2. **Take vitamin D_3 supplements.** Many scientists and experts recommend that you take a vitamin D_3 supplement each day. Depending on your age and current vitamin D_3 levels, you may want to supplement with 1000 to 4000 IUs daily. Speak to a specialist about the right dose for you. See tips #19 and #20 for advice on the best kind of supplements to buy.

3. **Eat foods rich in vitamin D_3.** Even though vitamin D_3 is not readily available in most foods, there are a few excellent sources. These include fatty fish, such as wild salmon, tuna and sardines, mushrooms and eggs.

19 Take the Right Kind of Supplements

If you decide to take supplements, it's important to know which kind to take. Not all supplements are the same quality, and many of the vitamins available on the market are synthetic and are made from petrochemicals, which really are not as efficient as natural sources. The problem is that the chemical compounds in synthetic vitamins are not found in nature and the human body finds it hard to recognize them and, as a result, to benefit from them. Moreover, when you get your nutrition from food, you get numerous vitamins and minerals from the same food source, and it is usually this complex combination of vitamins and minerals in the food that allows for proper nutrient absorption in the body. In other words, the vitamins and minerals in each food work together and interact for better absorption. For this reason, isolated vitamins, unless they are in the right combinations, don't have a salutary effect on the body, and they can even be treated like a toxin.

Water-soluble vitamins are flushed out of the body quite easily. But fat-soluble vitamins, such as vitamins A, D, E and K, accumulate and are stored in the body's fat tissues, fat deposits and liver, which makes the synthetic kind of fat-soluble vitamins potentially more toxic. So it's better to avoid the synthetic forms of these vitamins when possible. The many toxic ingredients found in these synthetic vitamins include magnesium stearate (stearic acid), "natural" flavors and sodium benzoate. Sodium benzoate is a preservative that kills everything alive in a product so it can sit on a shelf for weeks and months without spoiling. It is a known carcinogenic. Magnesium stearate suppresses the immune system and "natural" flavors contain MSG (monosodium glutamate).

Here are some tips for getting the most out of your vitamins:

- When shopping for vitamins, look for a range of supplements that are organic and made from 100 percent whole foods. These are processed without using excess heat, chemicals or harsh refining methods and therefore are more easily digested and absorbed by the body.

- Choose vitamins and minerals in a powdered form or in the form of natural oils or liquid concentrates as these are more easily absorbed by the body.

- Above all make sure that you eat a balanced, nutritious and varied diet of natural and organic foods, as that is the best and healthiest way to obtain the majority of your vitamins and minerals.

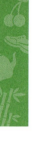

20 Get These Essential Vitamins and Minerals

Ideally, we'd get all our essential vitamins and minerals from the foods we eat and our environment. But depending on your diet, you may need to supplement with vitamins and minerals. Here's everything you need to know about taking supplements.

VITAMINS

Vitamins are essential for good health. Because your body does not create vitamins, you need to make sure that you get them from your food. If you are eating a healthy balanced diet consisting mainly of fruits and vegetables, preferably organic, then you are getting most of the vitamins and minerals your body needs. However, if you eat a lot of processed foods, conventionally grown fruits and vegetables and conventionally farmed animals, you might need to add food-based vitamins to your regimen.

There are two types of vitamins:

- **Fat-soluble vitamins** are stored in the fat tissues in your body and in your liver. They remain there until your body needs them. They include vitamins A, D, E and K.

- **Water-soluble vitamins** travel through your bloodstream and whatever your body doesn't need is excreted in your urine. These include B complex, vitamin C and folic acid.

When it comes to nutrients, the most important thing to do is to listen to your body. If you have a craving for a particular food, it's probably because you need the vitamin or mineral in it. If you decide to take a supplement, be aware that it often takes about two to four months for it to have any effect.

Here's a list of common vitamins, with their benefits and natural sources:

Vitamin A: Increase your vitamin A intake when you have problems with your skin, seem to get infections, find it hard to see in the dark or want to see color more clearly. Natural sources include eggs, fish, liver oil, liver, orange fruits and vegetables like cantaloupe, carrots and sweet potatoes, and dark green leafy vegetables like kale, collards and spinach.

Vitamin D: Increase your vitamin D intake to better absorb calcium and to develop strong bones. Vitamin D has been proven to alleviate depression, is administered as a preventative medicine against many serious illnesses and is also recommended if you have pain in your bones and muscle weakness. See tip #18 on vitamin D_3. Natural sources include eggs, oily fish and some fortified milk.

Vitamin E: Increase your vitamin E intake to improve blood circulation, protect your lungs from being damaged by air pollution and maintain your body's tissues. Natural sources are green leafy vegetables, nuts and seeds, egg yolks, sardines, wheat germ and whole grains.

Vitamin K: Increase your vitamin K intake if you have problems with blood clotting. Natural sources are leafy green vegetables, broccoli, milk, yogurt, cheese, eggs and meat.

Vitamin C: Increase your vitamin C intake when you are having problems with your gums or with nosebleeds, want to keep your muscles in good shape or have a wound or infection. Some natural sources of vitamin C are strawberries, tomatoes, broccoli, guavas, mangoes, cabbage, kiwi, red peppers, citrus fruits, cantaloupe, watermelon and papaya.

Vitamin B: The B vitamins are B_1, B_2, B_6, B_{12}, niacin, folic acid, biotin and pantothenic acid. Vitamin B is great to take if you want to increase your energy and improve your immune system. Vitamin B is commonly administered to those with a low red blood cell count (anemia) or an iron deficiency. Some good natural sources of vitamin B are meat, poultry, milk, yogurt, leafy green vegetables, beans, liver, nuts, wheat, oats and fish.

Folic Acid: If you have problems with anemia or are trying to get pregnant, you may want to take folic acid. Some good natural sources are spinach, green beans, cauliflower, brussels sprouts, whole grain breads, cereals, bean sprouts and broccoli.

MINERALS

Minerals are also vital for your body's functioning. They help to strengthen the skeleton, preserve the brain, transmit nerve impulses to make hormones and keep the heart healthy.

There are two kinds of minerals:

- **Macro Minerals:** Your body needs large amounts of macro minerals, which include calcium, iron and zinc.
- **Trace Minerals:** Your body needs trace minerals, but in smaller amounts than macro minerals. These include iodine, chromium and selenium.

Here's a list of essential minerals, with their benefits and natural sources:

Calcium: Take calcium to keep your bones and teeth strong and to support your nervous system. Good natural sources of it are dairy, leafy green vegetables and some fortified juices and cereals.

Iron: Take iron if you are anemic, meaning you have a low red blood cell count. Good natural sources of iron are meat, eggs, liver, dried fruits like raisins, fish and leafy green vegetables like broccoli and beans. Many iron supplements can cause constipation, so be sure to look for one that does not.

Zinc: Zinc really helps your immune function, so if you are susceptible to colds and flus, take this as a supplement. Zinc also is known to increase fertility, is essential for cell growth and helps heal wounds. Natural sources of zinc include milk, eggs, meat, leafy vegetables like broccoli, whole grains and the skin of baked potatoes.

Iodine: If you have problems with your thyroid, you may have an iodine deficiency. Iodine helps to metabolize excess fat. Natural sources of iodine are milk, fish, iodized salt, garlic, mushrooms and asparagus.

Chromium: Chromium helps maintain normal blood sugar levels. One in ten Americans is deficient in this mineral. Natural sources of chromium include meat, nuts, whole grains, corn oil and cloves.

Selenium: Selenium is an antioxidant that works in conjunction with vitamin E. It is found in Brazil nuts, brewer's yeast, broccoli, dairy, meat, grains and seafood.

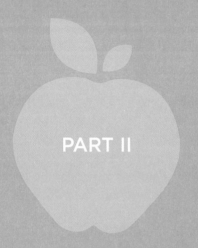

PART II

HEALTHY SELF

21 Look Younger from the Inside Out

There are many cosmetic ways to make you look younger from the outside in, but the following "inside out" solutions are much more powerful, long lasting and profound:

1. **Focus on the positive in people.** It's so easy to get frustrated with each other given the day-to-day stresses that we face, from misunderstandings to difficult personalities and poor communication. But rather than focus on the negative (the car that cut you off on the freeway), focus on the positive (the woman who let you in front of her at the checkout). The more loving and forgiving you are, the more relaxed and open your face will look.

2. **Let go now!** Release any built-up anger or frustration as quickly as possible. Holding on to these pent-up feelings is not only bad for your health, but it's certainly aging! Because anger is such a powerful emotion, often the only way to release it is through physical means. You may want to get a massage, bodywork, do some rigorous exercises or even attend an anger workshop to release this powerful emotion

from your cells. Once it's out you'll notice that your facial features soften and you look even younger.

3. **Focus on what you have.** The whole notion of and energy behind "wanting"—whether it's a new car, a bigger house, a better-paying job or anything else—can be very frustrating, and this longing and needing will inevitably show on your face. I call this the "when I have this or when I do this, then I will be happy" syndrome. It's great to have goals and dreams, but at the same time if you want to stay looking young, you need to appreciate the blessings you already have on a daily basis.

4. **Remember that you are not alone.** Whatever your religious or spiritual beliefs, you can benefit from strengthening your spiritual life and the sense that you are connected to all living things and are taken care of by a higher consciousness. This bigger connection will also help you to be aware of what your mission is here on the planet and how you make a difference. Knowing that you are making a difference in others' lives will automatically give your life meaning and take years off your face.

22 Stop These 3 Energy-Draining Habits

There are so many things that we do in our everyday lives that take up an exorbitant amount of unnecessary energy and drain our internal resources. Here are a few energy-draining habits to stop now:

Habit 1: Stop being so hard on yourself. Having high expectations for yourself is one thing, but having unreasonable expectations is another. With all your commitments and obligations, you may often feel like you want to be so many things to so many people so much of the time—especially to yourself. And when you're not able to do everything (as no one truly is), you may find that you are very hard on yourself rather than forgiving your limitations. If you can relax and let go of the need to be perfect, you will conserve your energy, be healthier and achieve so much more.

Habit 2: Embrace your demons. Maybe you have times when you feel envious, selfish or angry. So what! Put your hand in the air and cop to it. These feelings come and go and they are not who you are. There's something so self-accepting in recognizing that you don't have to be "good" all the time—it is okay to have negative emotions. Moreover, it's draining to try to stuff these negative feelings down and pretend that they don't exist. Instead, try to pinpoint the root cause of your feelings and address them. More often than not, fear is at the bottom of it all.

Habit 3: Stop judging others and being critical. It's too easy to get swept up in the latest gossip session and hop on the critical bandwagon. Don't give in! Instead, decide not to say a bad word about anybody. It will really help improve your energy, will make you feel more positive in general and will even make you more pleasant to be around. And keep in mind that when you talk badly of others, this reflects poorly on you—not the person you're talking about.

23 Express Your Feelings for Good Health

It is so easy to carry around unexpressed emotions, especially if you grew up in a family that didn't talk about their feelings or talk through disagreements. Bottling up your feelings and emotions is the biggest cause of hurt and upset feelings. Relationships break up over it and wars start because of it. However, if you can learn to communicate well, two individuals in their right mind can always come to an agreement. Here are some reasons why you want to express your feelings and emotions, rather than keep them bottled up inside:

1. **You will look younger.** Do you play out conversations with others in your head? If so, that is a sure sign that you have something to say and you need to say it. The bad news? An overload of negative internal chatter can create deep lines on your face and make you look older than you really are! So gather the courage and express what you need to, and you might find you look younger as the lines begin to soften.

2. **You will have less negative impact on your body.** Maybe you clench your jaw when you're angry, or you have a habit

of hunching your shoulders when you're stressed, as if you are carrying the weight of the world on your back. Whatever you do, these suppressed emotions have a way of lodging themselves internally and causing a negative impact on your body. If they remain unexpressed for a long period of time, they can really take their toll and ultimately cause long-term diseases, aches and pains. Once you get your thoughts and feelings off your chest, you'll notice the tension dissipate, along with your aches and pains.

3. **You will lose the tendency to exaggerate situations.** Unexpressed thoughts can often turn an issue into something bigger than it ever was intended or needed to be. If you mull over the original incident or conversation endless times in your mind, it has a tendency to twist and turn, and like in the game of telephone, it can easily change form, so that what the person said or did is totally different from what you think he or she said or did. Avoid turning a little incident into a stressful and unhealthy drawn-out drama by talking about it in the moment.

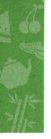

24 Listen to Calm Music and Sounds to Alleviate Stress

When you listen to music, it has a huge effect on your body. Fast sounds tend to energize you, quicken your heartbeat and increase your blood pressure. Slower, more instrumental music tends to help you de-stress, to slow your heartbeat, to lower your blood pressure, regulate stress hormones and elevate your mood.

Here are some bits of musical advice:

1. Be aware that the upbeat music playing in shops and supermarkets is intended to energize you and make you shop.
2. Classical music will help you relax after a hard day at work.
3. Play relaxing music before and after surgery to help you heal.
4. If you are a light sleeper, white noise can help by blocking out any distracting noises around you.
5. If you need help falling asleep, try listening to classical music or the sounds of nature, whether it is a babbling brook, ocean waves or raindrops.

25 Embrace Your Age

There is a moment in all our lives when the feeling that we are getting older hits us for the first time. It might be when you reach a significant age milestone, when you have a child or when you catch yourself in the mirror and see that those first lines have appeared on your face. But rather than dwell on the negative, being conscious of time moving forward can help you adopt healthy new habits.

1. **Recognizing Healthy Relationships:** Getting older makes you realize that your precious time is limited. So with that in mind, who would you like to spend more time with? Would you like to see certain members of your family more or allow a current friendship to develop to a new level?

2. **Leaving a Positive Legacy:** Getting older gives you a sense of urgency that will make you think deeply about what you are meant to be doing on the planet and how you want to leave a positive legacy behind. Not all of us have the opportunity to touch thousands of people's lives at once, in the way of a public figure. But it actually can be just as powerful and even

more meaningful to touch the lives of those around you: your family, your friends and your community. If you can make a difference in one person's life and give to them or teach them something, invariably they will pass it on to other people they come in contact with, and those others will hopefully, in turn, pass it on as well. So the effect of you making a difference is like a wave that radiates out and touches hundreds of people's lives without you knowing.

3. **Letting Go of Grudges:** Getting older makes you appreciate every moment of your life more. There is no time to waste on being at odds with anyone. If you have a disagreement, take the healthy route: let go of your ego and patch things up as quickly as you can. Give as much as you can to your family, friends and colleagues, especially when they least expect it, and when you come in contact with new people, think about what you can do for them, how you can help them, instead of what they can do for you.

26 Listen to Your Body

Have you noticed that when you get anxious or angry you suddenly get a physical ailment or even become accident-prone? Illnesses and accidents often occur at times of change or stress, such as moving to a new home, getting married or a change in your employment situation. This kind of uncertainty and fear can throw you off balance. In the same way, if you injure your body, you might want to look to see if there is a deeper, emotional component. Depending on the part of your body that is "stressed," this could mean different things:

Your Back: Your back represents your support system. If you tend to hold on to feelings or avoid dealing with them, you may experience back pain. If you do have back pain, ask yourself if you feel supported by those who are close to you. If you've had the pain for a while, think back to when it first started and see if you can remember whether you felt unsupported in your life when the pain began. Sorting out these old issues might help your back heal and release some of the stuck energy.

Your Arms: Your arms express your innermost feelings. Just think of all the things you do with your arms: holding, hugging, pushing away, folding to protect your heart, reaching out. Injuring your shoulder, elbow, wrist or hand can often be an indication of an emotional conflict and an ability to reach out to others.

Your Neck: Your neck gives you the ability to see all around you. When it becomes stiff, it limits your movement and vision. A stiff neck can indicate that you are becoming narrow in your views or do not want to look back or forward. If you do injure your neck, you might want to ask yourself, *What don't I want to look at?*

Your Legs: If you hurt your legs, often there is a conflict about the direction you are going in or a fear of moving forward.

Your Stomach: Your stomach is about digesting your reality, and not just your food. If your reality is indigestible, then indigestion can assail you. If you have a pattern of stomach issues, like acid in the stomach, stomach ulcers or constipation, you might want to determine if you are feeling emotionally nourished and if your reality is in conflict with what you really want.

27 Use Your Language to Help You Lose Weight

Many people don't realize how large a role language plays in their ability to lose weight or maintain a healthy weight.

For instance, most people have an innate fear of dying, so it is no wonder most of us struggle so hard with "die-ting." A word like that would scare even those with the best intentions in the world! The same goes for trying to "lose" weight. The word *lose* has a negative connotation to it. Nobody likes to "lose" anything, do they? So that's not the best choice of words. And that "weight" word...well, in this hypnotized, fast-food culture, where everyone hates "waiting" and would rather have everything now and deal with the consequences later, "weighting" doesn't cut it linguistically.

The everyday language that you use is really important and can really influence your personal habits. So become more conscious of your phrasing and choose language that is positive and enticing to help you achieve "optimum health."

The same goes for the way you communicate your intentions. How many times have you told yourself that you're going to start a diet "on Monday" or "next month" or "in the New Year"?

This sort of language that defers an action until some date in the future sends your body the wrong message. Rather than contemplating an exciting new life change, one that you could not possibly delay, as you want a healthy new you *now,* you imply that you're dreading this change so much that you will put it off until Monday, next month or the New Year. Success is much more achievable if you make a decision and take action immediately, and that usually happens when you are so sick of yourself, so fed up with how you feel and look, that you cannot "wait" (there's that word again) any longer and it has to happen now.

So the next time you feel motivated to change your life for the healthier, choose your words—and your intentions—carefully. They can make all the difference in your long-term success!

28. Stay Calm and Stress Free with These Easy Solutions

It has been estimated that 75 to 90 percent of visits to primary care physicians are for problems relating to stress, so obviously one of the best ways to stay healthy is to keep your stress levels low. Here are a few ways in which you can stay permanently calm regardless of what you are going through and what is going on around you:

1. **Change Your Language:** The everyday language that you use governs whether you see life as exciting or frightening, easy or hard, effortless or stressful. If you go through life as if it's a struggle and you wake up to "battle a new day" or you think people are "out to get you," your body is going to be in a heightened stress state, thinking that it is at war. Take the time to become a bit more conscious of the words that you use to describe your experiences, and choose words that relax you, rather than those that stress you out.

2. **Let Go of Tension:** Every now and again during the day check in with your body and notice where you are holding tension. Could your shoulders be more relaxed? Could your jaw loosen

its grip? Could you perhaps breathe a bit more deeply? If you are aware of where you hold your stress, you can direct your attention to those places in order to let it go.

3. **Find Happiness Independent of Achievement:** You have a sense of achievement when you reach your goals, which is separate from your ability to be happy and calm regardless of whether you have or haven't achieved what you think you desire. It's important to have goals in life, as it's exciting to work toward reaching them. But be a bit patient and don't let the fact that you might not have reached your goals yet suspend your ability to be happy and stress free every day. Be happy regardless of where you are on your journey, because if you are waiting to reach a goal before you enjoy your life—whether it's professional or personal—then one day you will look back and notice that you have wasted a lot of time.

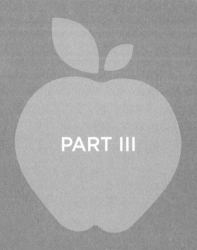

PART III

HEALTHY BODY

29 Combat the Winter Blues with These Simple Tips

Do the long, dark winters really get to you? Do you experience a serious mood change when the seasons change? Seasonal affective disorder (SAD) is a cyclic, seasonal condition. The signs and symptoms come and go at the same time every year and usually start appearing in the late autumn and go away during the sunny days of spring.

Here are some questions to pose to determine if you have SAD. In the winter, do you:

- Tend to eat more?
- Tend to sleep more?
- Put on more weight?
- Have less energy?
- Withdraw from friends?
- Feel more pessimistic?
- Have difficulty concentrating?
- Have an increase in anxiety?
- Generally feel a bit depressed?

If you answered yes to any of these, then you might have seasonal affective disorder. Here are some ways to combat SAD naturally:

1. Get as much sunlight as you can. Keep your curtains open, so your house and office are filled with light. Open your windows if the weather permits. Sit near windows as much as you can when you are at work, at home or on a bus so you can soak up the sun when it is out.

2. If it is sunny outside, regardless of how cold it is, bundle up and get some fresh air. Have lunch outside or take a walk, which can really lift your spirits.

3. Plan a vacation someplace warm in the winter so that you have something to look forward to and will have a break from the dark, cold weather.

4. Try a dawn stimulator or sunrise clock. It can be set like an alarm clock to produce an artificial gradual sunrise as you wake up in the morning.

5. Put an ionizer in the room that you spend most of your time in to keep the air fresh. Ionizers emit negative ions, which occur commonly in nature (for instance, after a rainstorm) and can create an overall sense of well-being and regulate hormone levels.

6. Plan activities in winter that keep your spirits lifted. Make sure you plan social engagements with people you like and whose company you enjoy, so that regardless of the weather, you are out and about with others.

7. Make sure that you have full-spectrum lights, which simulate natural light, in your home and office.

8. Try light therapy. Sit near a light box, a device that emits full-spectrum light but filters out ultraviolet rays for safety. Light boxes can mimic sunlight so that your body gets the benefits of the sun even during the dark winter months.

9. Make sure you maintain a healthy diet, take the vitamins and minerals that you need and exercise three to four days a week.

30 Exercise for Innumerable Benefits

One of the key ways to manage your weight and ensure good health on a long-term basis is to exercise at least three times a week. Most people who are not naturally inclined toward fitness need to find an incentive. Here are seven good reasons why you need to exercise:

1. Exercise significantly reduces your risk of illness and quickens your immune response.
2. Exercise helps you reach and maintain your ideal weight, so that you feel and look your best.
3. Exercise consistently leaves you in a better mood. Positive endorphins are released when you exercise, lifting your mood naturally.
4. Exercise may prevent injury over time by strengthening the muscles around the joints and keeping the joints in good working order. For instance, strengthening your core muscles through yoga or Pilates can decrease your risk of back injury.
5. Exercise helps you sleep better and gives you more consistent energy throughout the day.

6. Exercise improves your circulation and reduces your risk of muscle and bone loss as you age.
7. When you exercise, you set a good example for your partner, your children and the rest of your family.

If you think you don't have time to exercise, make time. Exercise needs to be part of your daily routine and it is a great way to either end your workday and transition to the evening or to kick-start your day in the morning. You can even squeeze in a workout during your lunch break.

The main key to sticking with exercise is to find a type that you enjoy. If the gym isn't for you, then find something physical that you do love. Try a yoga, a salsa or a kickboxing class, or some other exercise that you think will be fun. See what you enjoy and then just do it.

31 Practice Pilates for a Lean, Strong and Flexible Body

The Pilates method is a series of controlled movements that strengthen the core through the use of a range of apparatuses.

The goal of Pilates is to increase your strength, flexibility and control of your body. Pilates focuses on your breathing and your body alignment as you execute smooth, flowing movements. The emphasis is on the quality of the movements rather than the quantity. Controlled breathing helps you to use your body efficiently and release stress.

Unlike conventional workouts that are weight bearing and build short, bulky muscles, Pilates elongates your muscles, making them lean, strong and flexible. It improves your posture and makes you less prone to injury.

Pilates helps you develop a strong "core" at the center of your body. The core consists of the deep abdominal muscles, the muscles close to your spine and the trunk, pelvic girdle and shoulder girdle. Pilates conditions the whole body evenly, rather than overworking the same muscles and leaving others untouched, creating an imbalance.

Many sports teams and elite athletes use Pilates as part of their training regime. Physical therapy facilities utilize Pilates as a rehabilitation tool. It was originally used by ballet dancers and gymnasts and is still a critical part of their everyday training.

Pilates can help you:

- Recover from an injury and prevent one
- Increase your sports performance
- Improve your posture
- Become more fluid and supple
- Use your body more efficiently
- Improve your breathing
- Increase core strength and make you less prone to back injuries
- Engage your mind and enhance your awareness
- Become more mindful

Private Pilates classes are quite expensive, but it helps to have one-on-one instruction when you start out so that you learn the necessary techniques and avoid injury. Once you have a foundation, there are many group classes that you can partake in—check the offerings at your local gym, health center or Pilates studio.

32 Practice Yoga for Excellent Health

Yoga originated more than five thousand years ago in India, where it was seen as a complete mental and physical training to help one reach spiritual enlightenment. In recent years yoga has become extremely popular. There are many different types of yoga, and regardless of your age and fitness level, there is a type of yoga you will enjoy, whether it is a gentle exercise or a fast-paced, aerobic, sweat-filled workout. Yoga combines physical exercise and positions with breathing techniques and meditation. It can sharpen your mind and improve your emotional outlook.

In a yoga class, you are led through different poses, called asanas, and guided as to how to breathe throughout each series of poses. Don't be intimidated if the poses look difficult or if you don't think you are flexible enough to do them; with regular practice, your strength and flexibility will improve.

Here's some general advice if you are interested in practicing yoga:

- Start in a beginners' class, even if you are fit, because you will learn the basic yoga concepts and poses and proper alignment. What you learn from those beginning classes will carry you through your years of doing yoga and prevent you from getting injured.

- Find an instructor that adjusts your pose rather than just barks orders at the class. However, if the yoga teacher adjusts you in a position that feels unnatural and hurts, tell him or her to stop: you are in charge of your own body and you know its limits.
- Do not compare yourself to others in the class and force yourself beyond what you are capable of achieving. Be patient with yourself, because your body will loosen up over time. Remember that all great journeys begin at the beginning!

33 Be Smart about Antibiotics

Antibiotics are amazing, lifesaving substances when used properly. The problem is that we tend to overuse antibiotics these days, taking them at the first sign of a cold or other illness. Antibiotics only treat bacterial infections. They do not work against viruses. And if you take antibiotics when you don't need them, you will only weaken your immune system and become ill more often.

In addition to killing the unhealthy bacteria in your body, antibiotics also kill all the healthy bacteria. The good bacteria in your stomach is essential as it keeps your immune system strong, helps combat the unhealthy bacteria in your gut, aids digestion and provides essential nutrients and vitamins for your body.

You want to take antibiotics only when you really need them, and when you do, make sure you consume large amounts of probiotics simultaneously to replace the good bacteria in your gut.

34 Practice Reflexology on Yourself

Reflexology is based on the idea that different areas on the feet and hands correspond to different areas of the body, and that applying pressure to specific "reflex" areas with specific techniques can help move energy and improve the health of the corresponding body part. The concept behind reflexology is that there are small crystals of calcium and uric acid that accumulate around your reflex points, and by pressing and gently massaging the points through reflexology, you can break up the crystals and restore circulation and the energy flow.

Reflexology is not for treating potentially serious illnesses and is not a replacement for medical treatment. However, it is used in many hospitals and clinics in Europe and is known to be a very effective healing technique. Reflexology is said to speed healing, help eliminate toxins, improve circulation, lift your energy, relieve tension and headaches, and to help with stress, insomnia, PMS, constipation, back pain and eczema. The great thing about reflexology is that it is so easy to do on yourself when you are sitting at home, reading a book or watching TV.

Reflexologists believe that toxins are more likely to gravitate toward your feet, so focusing it on the reflex points on your feet can be more satisfying than working on your hands. Reflexology relieves tired feet after walking all day and squeezing into tight shoes. Here is how reflexology works:

1. Sit in a comfortable place where you can reach your feet easily.

2. To find the reflex points to focus on, refer to the reflexology chart on page 82. The right foot corresponds to the right side of the body and the left foot, to the left side.

   Alternatively, you can examine your feet to see which areas need attention. Move your thumbs from your toes to your heels, pressing all over your foot. The more tender any area is, the more out of balance it is—that is a reflex point for you to work on.

3. Once you have your reflex points, inch your thumbs along each point, applying slight pressure. You can stroke the area with your thumbs, make tiny circles or apply steady pressure on the point. Just take it slowly and gently and listen to your body. Think about using firm, steady pressure, so that the area is slightly tender, but not painful. As the calcium crystals and uric acid break up, you can go deeper.

4. Do each foot for five to fifteen minutes.

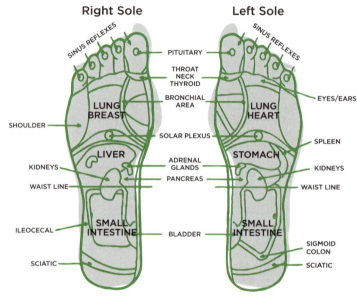

Reflexology points

35 Get a Regular, Inexpensive Massage

Massage has been around for thousands of years. It is perhaps the oldest therapy in the world. Experts estimate that about 90 percent of illnesses are stress related, and massage can help, as it is known to significantly reduce stress and relax the mind. The latest medical research shows that massage creates chemical changes that reduce pain and stress throughout the body.

Massage is one of the most popular forms of therapy in the world today. It is a simple and easy way to alleviate tension in our stressful lives and to create emotional, physical, mental and spiritual balance.

Regular massage is proven to help:

- Lower your heart rate
- Lower your blood pressure
- Improve your circulation
- Boost your immunity
- Improve digestion

- Increase your production of natural painkillers
- Speed your recovery from injuries
- Improve your sleep
- Improve your mood
- Better your concentration
- Alleviate depression

There are many different types of massage, including shiatsu, deep tissue, Swedish, sports massage and reflexology, to name a few. Depending on how hard or gentle you like your massage, you can easily find a type that suits you.

But don't think that you have to break the budget to get a massage! You can easily find a local salon that offers massages costing a dollar a minute. Or you can purchase a massage ball or personal massage machine to give yourself a massage, free of charge. Or try my personal favorite method: trade massages with your partner, a friend or a family member. I've even been known to pay my niece and nephew ten dollars each in exchange for a fifteen-minute massage!

36 Meditate

Stress is emotional and physical strain in response to pressure from the outside world. Any negative situation that causes you to make a rapid adjustment, such as arguing with your partner, your child or a friend, will cause stress, as will positive events, such as moving to a new house, changing jobs or getting married.

When you are under stress, your body reacts with the fight-or-flight response—your heart rate increases, your blood pressure rises and your breathing can become shallow and rapid. Your muscles and jaw tighten, you might sweat and your immune system becomes weaker as your physical and emotional tension soars. Stress can make you eat and drink too much, and can cause anxiety, depression, insomnia, muscle pain and skin rashes. The list of ailments triggered by stress is endless.

The way to healthily bring down your stress levels is to learn to relax and an easy way to do that is to take fifteen to twenty minutes out of your day to decompress: to control your breathing, relax your muscles and focus your mind. In other words, to meditate.

So many studies have shown the benefits of meditation. Among many things it can lower your blood pressure, improve your sleep, reduce chronic pain, calm your mind and leave you mentally alert, with increased energy.

There are many different meditation techniques and it is a matter of finding one that is good for you. Here is an exercise to get you started:

1. Find a quiet, comfortable place to sit, where you won't be interrupted for twenty minutes.

2. Pick a word with one or two syllables that helps you relax. Select *free, peace, quiet, love* or any other word that inspires you to *let go.*

3. Rest your hands on your lap, close your eyes and consciously relax your jaw and any other muscles that you notice are tight.

4. Silently repeat your word and keep repeating it. You may notice that your mind drifts off to events, work, family, people and other parts of your life. When you notice those thoughts, just acknowledge them, gently let them go and softly return to your word again. It doesn't matter if you have many thoughts and spend little time on your word. Just keep bringing yourself back to your word when you notice that your thoughts are drifting.

5. After twenty minutes, open your eyes. (You can check the time during the meditation by glancing at your watch while staying in your meditative state, or use a timer with a gentle ring to let you know that time is up.) When you have finished, take a few extra minutes to gently bring yourself back into the present moment by becoming aware of your body and how it feels and the sounds around you. When you are ready, continue with your day, refreshed, revitalized and full of life!

The ideal is to meditate twice a day, but even once a day is good for you. If you start practicing regularly, within a week or two you will see the benefits. In addition to dealing more easily with everyday obstacles and stresses, you'll probably find that you are calmer and more positive, that you sleep easier and that you have lower blood pressure!

37 Do Acupuncture

Acupuncture has been around for thousands of years and it really works. Acupuncture has to do with energy, or chi, in the body. Energy flows along pathways (meridians) in your body. Each pathway corresponds to one or a group of organs in the body. When illness or injury occurs, the chi backs up. If the chi is moving too fast or too slow, it can cause disease. The acupuncture needles are inserted along the meridian pathways, at points where the pathways are close to the surface of the skin. The needles release the chi to restore it to its normal flow and your symptoms are relieved as the chi moves smoothly around the body again.

The FDA considers acupuncture needles to be medical devices and they are regulated in the same way as other sterile medical equipment. Medical researchers have found that acupuncture stimulates your immune system and your nervous system to release endorphins, which are your body's natural painkiller. It also causes your body to release other natural chemicals, such as hormones, that regulate your body and control symptoms such as pain and swelling.

Here are just a few of the many ailments acupuncture can help with:

- Colds or flus
- Low energy or fatigue
- Sports injuries, such as a sprain or strain
- Allergies
- High blood pressure
- PMS
- Insomnia
- Depression and anxiety
- Asthma
- Infertility

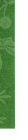

38. Use Acupressure for Common Ailments

Acupressure is based on the same concept as acupuncture (see tip #37), but without the needles. Instead of inserting needles, you apply pressure with your fingers and hands on meridian pathways to restore the normal flow of energy, or chi.

One of the best things about acupressure is that you can practice it on yourself. It is great for stress-related problems, like headaches, muscle aches, fatigue, insomnia, anxiety, motion sickness and constipation.

How to Do Acupressure

1. To massage an "acupoint," apply steady, firm pressure for about thirty seconds with your thumb, finger, elbow or palm.

2. Steadily press deeper for up to three minutes and then release and move on to your next point. If you can't reach an area (your back, for instance), you can lie on a massage ball or a tennis ball, but go easy. If the acupressure point is really sore, you want to go very slowly.

3. If you have difficulty locating an acupoint, move your fingers around the area until you find where it is sensitive.

There are many different acupressure solutions for common ailments. Here are four common ailments and ways to relieve the symptoms:

Headaches
Using the thumb and forefinger of one hand, pinch the webbed flesh between your thumb and forefinger (about an inch and a half in from the edge where the thumb and forefinger meet) of your other hand. Massage the point for two minutes. Then do the same on the other hand and repeat three times. This technique is also good for sinus ailments and toothaches.

Constipation and Indigestion
Put your right forefinger on top of your shin, just below your right knee, and then rest your other three fingers on your leg. Your pinkie will come to rest on a very powerful stomach point. When you press slightly, most likely the area will feel sensitive. Press firmly for one minute, take a break and do this three more times. Change to the left leg.

Hangovers
I thought I might throw this one in, as many suffer from these!

Do small circular movements on top of your foot two finger widths down from your ankle and between your big toe and the second toe. It will feel tender. Apply pressure here with deep strokes. This technique is also good if you have sore feet!

PMS and Menstrual Cramps

There are a few points that relieve these symptoms. This is an easy one. On the inside of your leg, measure three or four finger widths up from the ankle toward the knee. You will notice that this area is tender. Apply pressure for a minute and then release. Do this three times and repeat as needed.

39 See a Chiropractor for Back Pain

Eight out of ten people suffer from some form of back pain in their lifetime, due either to poor muscle tone, bad posture, athletic or other injuries, disk problems, or a problem in the legs or buttocks. Emotional stress, long periods of inactivity, repetitive strain and heavy physical work can also cause back pain.

If you do have back pain, I suggest that you do not rush to a medical doctor. Instead, visit a chiropractor. Chiropractic is the third largest doctoral-level health profession, after medicine and dentistry. It is covered by most insurance policies and addresses lower back pain, neck problems, headaches and other chronic pain, and all sorts of athletic injuries.

Chiropractic is a system of therapy that returns the body to a balanced state by manipulating the spine and joints to restore normal motion and reduce any nerve interference. Many diseases are connected to poor alignment of the vertebrae. Chiropractors treat disease by manipulating the vertebrae in order to relieve pressure on the nerves.

Chiropractors are extremely well trained, so you can feel confident in a chiropractor's hands. If they can't help you, they will let you know and will recommend that you consult a medical doctor. Finding the right doctor of chiropractic is just as important as finding the right dentist or medical doctor. It is best to get a recommendation from a friend or medical professional. You may even be able to get a referral through your health insurance.

40 Do the Alexander Technique

A medical doctor first recommended that I do the Alexander technique when I was fourteen and suffering from a back injury. Not only did it help my back, but it also taught me how to sit, stand, lift objects and walk with so much more ease. Even today people ask about my good posture, and it's all thanks to my training in the Alexander technique.

The basic idea of the Alexander technique is to get rid of tension in the body, correct the misuse of muscles and change bad alignment habits in your everyday activities, for example, when you are sitting, lying down, standing, walking or lifting something. The goal is to improve your ease and freedom of movement and learn the proper way to perform different activities, without causing any strain on your body.

Alexander reeducates the mind and body and is one of the most popular techniques used by actors, singers and musicians, because it helps the performer relax onstage and use the least amount of energy for movement. I highly recommend the Alexander technique for everyone, because not only will it help you let go of unhealthy habits, but it will improve your posture and hence your confidence.

If you feel that your posture can be improved or that you carry stress unnecessarily in any part of your body, if you have a bad back or neck, or simply want to understand more on how your body is meant to move or aim to protect it from repetitive strains, then the Alexander technique is for you.

41 Stock Your Homeopathic Medicine Cabinet

Homeopathy is a system of natural health care that has been employed worldwide for over two hundred years. It is recognized by the World Health Organization as the second largest therapeutic system in the world.

The concept is that you treat the patient, not the disease, on all levels: spiritual, emotional, mental and physical. The overriding principle in homeopathy is that you treat "like with like," meaning the remedies produce the same symptoms as the illness to counteract and cancel them out. Substances that cause symptoms similar to those of the ailment are highly diluted and taken with the aim of activating the body's natural healing system. For example, drinking too much coffee can cause sleeplessness, agitation and even palpitations, and the homeopathic remedy *Coffea* can treat all these problems.

There are many qualified homeopaths that you can go to for very personalized treatment. You can easily treat common, everyday illnesses yourself with homeopathic remedies. You can find them in most drugstores and in health food stores. These remedies are safe and nontoxic, and as there are no side effects, they can be given to anyone, from babies to pregnant women and the elderly. They are a great complement to standard medical treatment and are often recommended by medical doctors who know about homeopathy.

Here are a few remedies that you might want to have available in your medicine cabinet:

Aconite-Good for fevers, colds and flus, as well as for panic attacks and a variety of minor childhood illnesses, such as earache, sore throat, flu and fever.

Arnica-Soothes sore muscles, bumps and bruises.

Arsenicum-Good for nausea, vomiting, diarrhea and food poisoning.

Belladonna-Good for sore throats, headaches, earaches, fever, heartburn, gas, bloating and upset stomach.

Hypericum-In cream form, it is good for pain and infection in cuts, scrapes and stings. Used internally, it is good for nerve pain and backaches.

Nux Vomica-Good for motion sickness and hangovers. It can relieve nausea, vomiting, fatigue, headaches, cramps, heartburn, ulcers, hiccups and constipation.

Rhus Tox-Good for rashes and itching. It is diluted poison oak and is a great remedy for poison ivy and eczema.

42 Do Traditional Chinese Medicine

Traditional Chinese medicine (TCM) dates back five thousand years. Unlike in Western medicine, where doctors focus on the body part giving you trouble, in TCM your body is seen as an integrated web of systems that can get out of balance, and health problems arise when your flow of energy, or chi, is blocked. TCM emphasizes healing with herbs, diet, *Tui Na* massage and acupuncture. Tai chi and *Qigong* are also closely associated.

TCM uses the opposing forces of yin and yang as the fundamental way of understanding the body and health. Yin and yang represent dark and light, male and female, hot and cold. When yin and yang get out of balance, you get sick. There are five different changing aspects within yin and yang, which need to be in harmony: Earth, Fire, Metal, Water and Wood. Each interacts with the other in a complex system.

TCM can be helpful for many health problems, such as chronic pain, allergies, colds and flus, skin conditions, digestive problems, infertility and lack of energy.

As part of the initial exam, the TCM doctor will check your pulse and look at your tongue. The color and shape of your tongue give the doctor an insight into the health of your internal organs, as each part of your tongue correlates to an area or organ in your body.

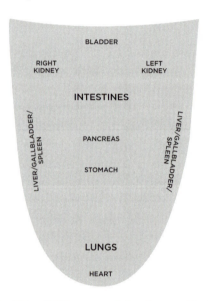

Traditional Chinese medicine tongue chart

43 Use Fluoride-Free Toothpaste and Mouthwash

Fluoride is in virtually every brand of toothpaste, and many experts claim that it helps to fight tooth decay. However, this chemical has been linked to many health issues, including cancer. In 2007, researchers found that children living in communities with fluoridated water had elevated lead levels, which may explain the corrosion in the pipes. Dr. John Lee, a fluoride toxicity researcher, has established a direct link between fluoride use and osteoporosis, and a growing number of doctors and researchers are expressing concern about the public's exposure to fluoride in the water. Fluoride compounds that are put in the water supply to fight tooth decay, in toothpaste and in supplement tablets have never been tested for safety.

In fact, if you read the back of most toothpastes you will notice a sign warning you to keep the toothpaste away from children under six years of age and to contact a poison control center if accidentally swallowed. Since 1997, the U.S. Food and Drug Administration has mandated that all toothpastes containing fluoride carry this warning.

Statistics also show that there is no difference in the dental health of children who use fluoride and those who don't.

In addition to fluoride, most commercial toothpastes contain substances that are hazardous when swallowed, such as paraben, petroleum, synthetic flavorings, synthetic fragrance, mineral oil, propylene and glycol.

To limit your exposure to fluoride, filter your home water (choose a filter that removes fluoride) and opt for natural, fluoride-free toothpaste and mouthwash.

44 Buy Toxin-Free Cosmetics

Unlike the food and drug industry, there is little regulation when it comes to cosmetic and beauty products. As a result, many cosmetic and beauty products contain toxic ingredients, because they are considered inexpensive and ensure a long shelf life. These ingredients include coal-tar colors, phenylenediamine, benzene and formaldehyde—believe me, nothing you'd want to put in your body!

Unfortunately for your health, these potentially harmful chemicals are absorbed into the body and can get into the bloodstream in many different ways. Hair sprays, perfumes and powders are inhaled, eye makeup is absorbed by mucous membranes and lipstick can be swallowed. (Apparently, on average, women eat four to seven pounds of lipstick in their lifetime!) And shampoos, hair dye, conditioners, body creams and blush are all absorbed through the skin.

Here are three things you can do to protect your health where cosmetics are concerned:

1. Read the labels to make sure that your makeup has natural and organic ingredients, made from botanicals and natural

minerals, colored clays and vegetable oils. You are looking for makeup that contains ingredients that you recognize from nature. By rule of thumb, if you can't pronounce a name on the ingredients list, it probably isn't good for you.

2. If you don't know what an ingredient is in a product, look it up before you buy it. Often the ingredient names are code for hidden ingredients. For example, the word *fragrance* is often used to refer to the many chemicals in a fragrance. *Talc* sounds safe, but it is actually similar to asbestos, and parabens are preservatives that increase the shelf life of products but are known to be toxic. You will notice that many healthier products will mention that they are paraben free on the label!

3. If in doubt, go light on the makeup. A more natural look is very appealing—perhaps just shape your eyebrows nicely, put on some mascara, wear a little bit of lip gloss and a dab of powder where you need it.

45 Get Beautiful, Natural Nails

Many people don't think twice about the kind of polish they use on their nails, but the truth is, your nails are porous, and your nail polish may not be as healthy as you think. There are no requirements to list nail polish ingredients on the label, so you have no way of knowing what dangerous chemicals are in it. In fact, most nail polishes contain a substantial amount of phthalates and formaldehyde, which are thought to be carcinogenic.

There are seven very simple actions that you can take to make sure that your porous nails are not absorbing dangerous chemicals into your body.

1. Purchase water-based nail polish from your local health food store; in these the chemical solvents are replaced by water.

2. Acetone is a powerful solvent and actually strips the nails. As an alternative, use a non-acetone nail polish remover. It takes longer but is much healthier for you.

3. Try to avoid using acrylic nails, as they can easily rip off a layer of your natural nail when removed.

4. If you can, stay away from polish altogether. It's still possible to get a polished look by doing your own manicure: shape and buff your nails and use a nourishing cuticle oil.

5. Strong nails start with a really healthy diet, so be sure you're getting all the necessary nutrients from your food.

6. If you are pregnant or breast-feeding, the safest option is to leave your nails alone. If you do want to polish your nails, use water-based polish.

7. If you go to a salon, make sure that it is clean and they are disinfecting their tools in between customers so that you aren't exposed to harmful germs or bacteria.

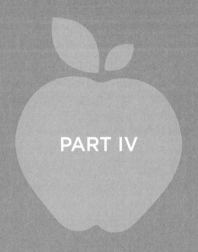

PART IV

HEALTHY EARTH

46 Avoid BPAs

An expert panel of researchers has found that plastic made with a chemical called bisphenol A (commonly known as BPA) is highly toxic and can easily leach into your food and drink. It is known to act as an endocrine disrupter in that it mimics the effect of estrogen in the body. Research has shown that exposure to BPA puts you at greater risk of developing uterine fibroids and breast cancer and can cause a decrease in sperm count and early onset of puberty in exposed children.

BPA is widely used in the manufacture of baby bottles, drinking bottles, oven and microwave dishes, eating utensils and is even in the plastic coating inside metal cans. Here are some dos and don'ts regarding plastics, including those with BPA:

1. Avoid heating food in plastic containers. When plastic is heated or stressed, it releases small amounts of its ingredients. So BPA can leak out depending on the temperature of the food and liquid.

2. Do not microwave your food in plastic containers. Instead use glass, such as Pyrex, or ceramic containers for heating food.

3. Avoid canned food and drinks, as the lining of many tins contains BPA.
4. Do not wash plastic containers in the dishwasher.
5. Get rid of any scratched plastic containers.
6. Make sure that your water bottles are BPA free. Use a glass or stainless-steel water bottle rather than plastic when you can. (Just make sure that it is stainless steel inside and out.) When you wash your water bottle, always let it dry before you refill it to keep bacteria away.
7. Make sure that you buy baby bottles, sippy cups and children's tableware that are BPA free. The package will say "BPA free."
8. Avoid any food containers with the number 3 or 7 on the recycling label on the bottom, as most of them contain BPA and other dangerous substances. (Food containers 1, 2 and 4 do not contain BPAs.) See tip #47 for more details.

47 Know Which Plastics Are Safe to Use

So many everyday items that you use are made of plastic, including food containers, drink containers, children's toys and kitchen utensils. You are surrounded by plastic in one form or another! Because it is used in so many different ways, it is important to know which plastic is safe for you, your family and the earth.

Plastics do not biodegrade and consequently constitute 90 percent of all trash floating in the world's oceans.

Research shows that some plastics are toxic or cause hormonal changes in the body. Studies have also shown that fish and birds are experiencing hormone disruption because of plastic: the sea is thick with dangerous synthetic particles.

How do you know which plastic is the safest kind to choose? Every time you buy or use a plastic container, turn it upside down and look at the bottom. There you will find a number between one and seven inside a recycling symbol. This number tells you what kind of plastic the container is made out of, whether it can be recycled or not and whether it is hazardous to your health or not. Here is a guide to what the numbers mean. You'll notice that numbers 3 and 7 are the most dangerous.

1. **Polyethylene Terephthalate (PET or PETE):** This is generally considered safe and is used to make soft drink, water, sports drink, ketchup and salad dressing bottles. It is not known to leach any chemicals that are suspected of causing cancer or disrupting hormones. However, it does have a porous surface on which bacteria can grow, so you should never reuse this bottle.

2. **High-density Polyethylene (HDPE):** This is generally considered safe. It is used to make milk, water and juice bottles, butter and yogurt containers, cereal box liners and trash bags. It is not known to leach any unhealthy chemicals.

3. **Polyvinyl Chloride (PVC):** This is unsafe. It is used to make plastic food wrap, frozen dinner containers, bottles for cooking oil and plumbing pipes. PVC is tough plastic, and to make it flexible, manufacturers add "plasticizers" during production. Traces of these chemicals can leach out of PVC when in contact with foods. They are suspected human carcinogens. Avoid microwaving with plastic wrap as the high heat causes the poisonous toxins to melt out of the plastic wrap and to drip onto the food.

4. **Low-density Polyethylene (LDPE):** This is generally considered okay. You will find it in some bread and frozen food bags, squeezable bottles and grocery bags. It is not known

to leach any dangerous chemicals, but it is also not generally accepted for recycling.

5. **Polypropylene (PP): This is generally considered okay.** You will find it in some ketchup bottles, yogurt containers, margarine tubs and medicine bottles. It is hazardous during production but is not known to leach any chemicals. It is increasingly being accepted for recycling.

6. **Polystyrene (PS), or Styrofoam: This is unsafe.** You will find this in disposable plates and cups, containers and packaging, and toys. There is much evidence to suggest that this type of plastic leaches potentially toxic chemicals, especially when heated. It is also very difficult to recycle.

7. **Everything Else (usually polycarbonate, including BPA): This is unsafe.** The number refers to all other types of plastics, including BPA, or plastics made with bisphenol A. BPA is a hormone disruptor and is highly toxic. (See tip #46 for more information.) It is found in baby bottles, food storage containers, computer cases, microwave oven ware, eating utensils and the plastic coating in metal cans. It can leach into food as the product ages and with a temperature change and is very difficult to recycle.

48. Use Your Cell Phone Safely

Cell phones are extremely convenient and most people seem to have them. In fact, according to the International Telecommunication Union (ITU) five billion of the seven billion people on the planet currently have mobile phone subscriptions.

On the downside, cell phones emit electromagnetic fields (EMFs) and their safety is continuously being debated. Some studies show that cell phones are safe, yet other studies show that prolonged use of cell phones can expose you to damaging levels of radiation—and that we may be facing an epidemic of brain tumors as a result.

While the research isn't clear yet, it's important to remember that cell phones have been popular only for a short time, and it can often take decades for cancers to develop. If you look back at the history of the cigarette industry, you will recognize that it took decades to prove that cigarettes were bad for your health. So as we continue to learn more about the effects of this new technology, here are some ways in which you can lower your potential health risk and err on the side of caution:

1. Use your cell phone as little as possible, and if you must use it, keep your talk time down to a real minimum.

2. Be aware of how the side of your head and your ear feel when you use your phone. If you feel any heat or a slight throbbing, end the call, transfer your call to a landline or tell the caller you will call back from a landline.

3. Do not carry your phone on your person. You do not want to hang it round your neck, place it near your heart, put it in your pocket or clip it to a belt, place it near your genitals or even hold it in your hand for long periods. The phone continuously emits radiation and it will affect any organ or part of your body that it is close to or touching. When you can, put the phone on your desk or in your bag or purse, away from your body.

4. By far the best method if you have to use a cell phone is to use the speaker phone and be hands free, making sure that you keep the actual phone as far away from you as possible. This is easy to do in a car as you can easily feed the phone through a speaker system and keep the phone about a foot away from you at the same time.

5. Use your phone when it has the best reception, because when the reception is good, the phone emits less radiation. When the reception is bad, the phone uses more power and emits

more radiation to try and get a signal. You want the phone to operate on as little power as necessary. So do not cover the receptor with your hand while you speak, and if you notice that the reception is poor, move to an area with better reception before taking or making a call.

6. Wearing an earpiece headset like a Bluetooth exposes you to less radiation than the cell phone does, but it still emits radiation, so do not wear it all the time. When you do use the Bluetooth, make sure your calls are short and you regularly switch the ear you have the piece on.

7. There are many reasonably priced products on the market that can protect you from the radiation emitted by your cell phone, such as a cell phone EMF shield, an Air Tube Earpiece and snap-on ferrite beads.

8. Children are more susceptible to radiation damage than adults, so let them use a cell phone only in emergency situations or very infrequently.

49. Clean Your Home Naturally—and Healthily

Many of the cleaning products that you keep in your kitchen cupboards, underneath your sink and in the bathroom cabinets are extremely toxic and hazardous to your health. These products are dangerous if inhaled and if they come in contact with your skin, and can be deadly if swallowed.

The good news is that in recent years many ecological cleaning products have come on the market that are much safer than the toxic commercial products. Rather than expose yourself to toxic chemicals regularly, it makes much more sense to replace the old, hazardous products with environmentally friendly products. The environmental ones might be slightly more expensive, but it is definitely worth the extra cost to limit the amount of toxins that you expose yourself and your family to.

If you want to make the transition easy, then swap out one product at a time, exchanging the commercial products for the ecological ones as you run out. If you think that ecological cleaning products are too pricey, here are three inexpensive, safe, easy and more natural alternatives to try:

1. **Use white distilled vinegar.** This is really effective as a general household cleaner as it has a very high level of acidity, which helps to kill bacteria, mold and germs. It is very environmentally friendly and inexpensive.

2. **Use baking soda.** This is great for cleaning because it has the ability to dissolve dirt and grease in water. It is completely natural, maintains a pH balance and eliminates odors. It's perfect for cleaning kitchen and bathroom countertops and eliminating odors from the fridge, garbage disposal, trash cans and the dishwasher. You can even sprinkle it on the carpet to fight pet and other odors.

3. **Use cornstarch.** This is great for soaking up grease and oil stains. You can use it to clean countertops, remove stains from carpets and it works very well as a window cleaner. It is also great as an ironing aid and is much better to use on your baby than baby powder.

50 Improve Your Indoor Air Quality

According to the Environmental Protection Agency (EPA), the average American home is hundreds of times more polluted inside than out, and exposure to air pollutants in the home and office can cause significant health risks. At any one time you can be exposed to viruses, bacteria and mold; chemical fumes from formaldehyde in the carpets, furniture, paint and bedding; and particles in the air, such as allergens, dust and pollen—to name but a few!

You might need an air purifier to protect yourself and your family, especially if any of you suffer from asthma, immune illnesses, fatigue, headaches or respiratory illnesses. The best device for cleaning indoor air is a HEPA (high-efficiency particulate air) filtration unit.

Here are a few additional tips to improve your air quality:

1. Buy a portable air filtration unit to put inside your home.
2. Take your shoes off at the door so that you limit the amount of toxins you bring in from outside.

3. Air out any new carpeting or furniture so that the toxins from the paint or chemicals do not affect your health.

4. If you have children, limit their exposure to plastic toys, which might contain hazardous materials.

5. Most rugs and carpets contain formaldehyde, so make sure you have plants to soak up the toxicity. If you have the choice, go formaldehyde free.

6. Change your conventional cleaning products and air fresheners to environmentally friendly ones (see tip #49).

7. Sick on a regular basis? Have your house tested for mold.

8. Open your windows regularly to let in fresh air and to improve the quality of the air in the house.

9. Do not smoke inside the home.

10. Use more natural and organic personal care products instead of toxin-filled commercial kinds (see tips #44 and #45).

SO, HOW HAPPY *IS* YOUR HEALTH?

Now it's time to find out how happy your health really is—and how you can make it even happier. Take your quiz responses and follow the suggestions below to see which tips will help you create a happier, healthier and longer life.

1. **If you answered:**
   A. See tips: 1, 48
   B. It's great that you are aware that it is better to speak from a landline whenever possible. Now read on for additional tips to help you become even healthier.
   C. See tips: 1, 48

2. **If you answered:**
   A. See tips: 2, 46, 47
   B. It's great that you are aware of the quality of the water that you drink. Now read on for additional tips to help you become even healthier.
   C. See tips: 2, 46, 47

3. **If you answered:**
    A. See tips: 49, 50
    B. Congratulations on being so mindful of what toxins you have in your home. Now read on for additional tips to help you become even healthier.
    C. See tips: 49, 50

4. **If you answered:**
    A. It's great that you are aware that your body absorbs whatever you put on it. Now read on for additional tips to help you become even healthier.
    B. See tips: 43, 44, 45, 49
    C. See tips: 43, 44, 45, 49

5. **If you answered:**
    A. See tips: 46, 47
    B. It's good that you are aware of the potential toxic effects of plastic. Now read on for additional tips to help you become even healthier.
    C. See tips: 46, 47

6. **If you answered:**
   A. See tips: 1, 2, 3, 12, 13, 15, 16, 19, 20, 30, 31, 32, 34, 35, 37, 38, 39, 40, 41, 42
   B. It's good that you know how to look after yourself and take care of your own body. Now read on for additional tips to help you become even healthier.
   C. See tips: 1, 2, 3, 12, 13, 15, 16, 19, 20, 30, 31, 32, 34, 35, 37, 38, 39, 40, 41, 42

7. **If you answered:**
   A. It's great that you are conscious of your posture and how it affects your health, well-being and confidence! Now read on for additional tips to help you become even healthier.
   B. See tips: 31, 32, 35, 36, 39, 40
   C. See tips: 31, 32, 35, 36, 39, 40

8. **If you answered:**
   A. It's fortunate that you are not particularly moody. Now read on for additional tips to help you become even healthier.
   B. See tip: 29
   C. See tips: 21, 22, 23, 24, 25, 28, 30

9. **If you answered:**
   A. See tips: 30, 31, 32, 39
   B. It's excellent that you are conscious that exercise is a big part of living a healthy life. Now read on for additional tips to help you become even healthier.
   C. See tips: 30, 31, 32

10. **If you answered:**
    A. See tips: 10, 11, 12, 14, 15, 16, 17, 27, 30
    B. It's very smart that you take care of yourself consistently and do not feel the need to diet. Now read on for additional tips to help you become even healthier.
    C. See tips: 2, 10, 11, 12, 14, 15, 16, 17, 27, 30

11. **If you answered:**
    A. You know that if you take care of your body, it will take care of you. Now read on for additional tips to help you become even healthier.
    B. See tips: 1, 2, 3, 4, 5, 6, 7, 8, 9, 12, 13, 14, 15, 16, 17, 18, 19, 20, 21, 22, 23, 24, 25, 26, 28, 30, 31, 32, 33, 34, 35, 36, 37, 38, 39, 40, 41, 42, 43, 44, 45, 46, 47, 48, 49, 50

C. See tips: 1, 2, 3, 4, 5, 6, 7, 8, 9, 12, 13, 14, 15, 16, 17, 18, 19, 20, 21, 22, 23, 24, 25, 26, 28, 30, 31, 32, 33, 34, 35, 36, 37, 38, 39, 40, 41, 42, 43, 44, 45, 46, 47, 48, 49, 50

12. If you answered:
  A. See tips: 21, 22, 23, 24, 25, 28, 30, 32, 34, 35, 36, 37, 38, 40
  B. You are very lucky that you have a calm disposition and that very few things stress you out; that is a big key to health. Now read on for additional tips to help you become even healthier.
  C. See tips: 21, 22, 23, 24, 25, 28, 30, 32, 34, 35, 36, 37, 38, 40

13. If you answered:
  A. It's great that you do not equate reaching your goals with happiness. Now read on for additional tips to help you become even healthier.
  B. See tips: 21, 22, 25, 28
  C. See tips: 21, 22, 25, 28

14. If you answered:
  A. It's very healthy that you can easily release anger and don't hold grudges. Now read on for additional tips to help you become even healthier.

- **B.** See tips: 21, 22, 23, 25, 26, 28
- **C.** See tips: 21, 22, 23, 25, 26, 28

15. If you answered:
- **A.** See tips: 10, 11, 12, 17
- **B.** It's fantastic that you consciously eat to sustain energy and you think of the long-term effects. Now read on for additional tips to help you become even healthier.
- **C.** See tips: 10, 11, 12, 16, 17

16. If you answered:
- **A.** See tips: 19, 20
- **B.** See tips: 19, 20
- **C.** It's terrific that you are aware that there is a difference in the quality of vitamins and minerals available. Now read on for additional tips to help you become even healthier.

17. If you answered:
- **A.** It's great that you see the benefit of eating organic. Now read on for additional tips to help you become even healthier.
- **B.** See tips: 3, 4, 5, 19
- **C.** See tips: 3, 4, 5, 19

18. If you answered:

A. It's excellent that you reach for something healthy when you want to snack. Now read on for additional tips to help you become even healthier.

B. See tips: 11, 12, 15, 17

C. See tips: 11, 12, 15, 17

19. If you answered:

A. It's great that you are aware of the quality of animal products that you buy. Now read on for additional tips to help you become even healthier.

B. See tips: 3, 6, 7, 8, 9

C. See tips: 3, 6, 7, 8, 9

20. If you answered:

A. See tips: 3, 4, 5, 6, 7, 9, 12, 13, 14, 16

B. It's extremely beneficial that you eat a diet rich in healthy fruits and vegetables. Now read on for additional tips to help you become even healthier.

C. See tips: 1, 2, 3, 4, 5, 6, 7, 8, 9, 10, 11, 12, 13, 14, 15, 16, 17, 18, 19, 20

ACKNOWLEDGMENTS

I would like to thank the countless wonderful doctors, health practitioners, therapists, self-development trainers and environmentalists, who have in one way or another contributed to this book. From my early teens, each one of you over time has assisted to help open my eyes to what real health means and have influenced the way that I treat my body and consequently the knowledge that I impart about such topics as the food that we eat, the toxins we ingest, how we holistically can heal our bodies and how the mind and spirit have a deep influence on the body. I would like to extend a special public thanks to Dr. Yamamoto, Professor Larry, Dr. DeAndrea, John Wood, Dr. Hakhamimi, Ty Thornton and HRH the Prince of Wales.

Thank you to my exceptional editor, Sarah Pelz, and the rest of the team at Harlequin, who have and continue to work so hard on the *How Happy Is* book series. A special thanks also go to Tara Kelly and Mark Tang for joining forces with the book design, as well as Shara Alexander and the rest of the marketing team.

My fantastic book agent's Shannon Marven, Lacy Lynch, Jan Miller and everyone at Dupree Miller—thank you for pulling my book proposal out of the slush pile twice! It was obviously meant to be and proves that every now and again cold calling can work!

Thanks to the *Huffington Post,* Babette Perry, Wendy Cohen, Joel Mandel and Scott Warren for your support. Thanks also go to Sam Fischer and P.J. Shapiro for watching my back, and Ashley Davis and Andrea Ross, my agents at CAA.

Thanks also to my colleagues at HowHappyIs.com, especially Jon Stout for his endless creativity, Terri Carey for keeping us organized and Serena Zanello for her illustrations.

To my lovely aunt, Evonne, for being ahead of her time when it came to alternative medicines and eating organic. While everyone laughed and called us "mad," we did it anyway.

Oli, the love of my life, and Judah, the happiest boy, you rock!

Look for these other books in the *How Happy Is* series!

How Happy Is Your Love Life?

How Happy Is Your Marriage?

How Happy Is Your Home?